AF200322

D r. S t e f a n B r o s i g

Ginger, Horseradish and Licorice in Horse Feeding

Foods as effective medicines

additionally

Mosses against fungal diseases

Ambulant treatment of keratoma

Glued-on dressings on wounds

Treatment of cracks in hooves

Use of ginger and horseradish in humans

The author has a Ph.D. in physical chemistry, rides since 1978 and owns horses since 1986

Bibliographic information of Die Deutsche Bibliothek for the German edition:

Die Deutsche Bibliothek lists the German publication in the Deutsche Nationalbibliographie; detailed bibliographic data can be recalled via internet: <http://dnb.ddb.de>

Copyright 2018 Dr. Stefan Brosig
Copyright (German edition) 2006 2008 2010 2013 Dr. Stefan Brosig
Production and publishing: BoD- Books on Demand, Norderstedt
German edition ISBN: 978-3-8334-6928-2
English language edition ISBN: 978-3-7481-7142-3
Cover design: Anja Küstner, Jörg Endrich, Stefan Brosig
Photos: Stefan Brosig, Elke von Lingelsheim, Imke Eppers

This book is dedicated to my warmblood gelding and former riding-school horse Waran (1971 – 2006), for whom ginger, and later on horseradish, was the first to extend his life in a beautiful and liveable way!

On the day of his death a poem came into my mind spontaneously, which I have cited here in German, as I find no fitting English words to translate it. But the translation of the title is "Farewell".

Abschied

Lange waren wir beisammen,
haben vieles schon erlebt,
war'n uns liebe Kameraden,
bis zuletzt die Stunde schlägt!

Durch das Leben schwach geworden,
gib mich frei und laß mich zieh'n!
Keine Trennung ist auf Dauer,
bald schon gibt's ein Wiederseh'n!

Und bis dahin, sei nicht traurig,
besser könnt' es mir nicht geh'n!
Mit den Freunden, die schon gingen,
ewig jung und ewig kräftig,
immer gut gelaunt und prächtig,
über ewiggrüne Weiden,
lüftetrinkend, jag' ich hin!

(written on July 30th 2006)

Foreword to the English translation of the 4th German edition

At first I want to apologize for the long time I needed to present an English translation of my book which has already proved so valuable to many horse-owners in Germany! Ginger has been elected medicinal plant of the year 2018 in Germany and this gave an additional motivation to get it finally done! Although as a scientist I have to be able to read English fluently, the active usage is a bit "hampered".... Thus I also want to apologize in advance for translation mistakes, which you will surely find when reading it. But the described treatments itself should nevertheless be described clearly enough, as I believe. With a little help by a Pittsburgh lady I could at least erase some very big blunders!

In the English version of the 4th German edition I have omitted some treatments, which have now become unnecessary since there are in the meantime enough other effective treatments on the market. These omitted treatments concern the prevention of crib-biting and treatment of thrush.

I also want to point out that the most important thing always is the removal of the causes of maladies!

In this respect I also want to point to a VERY important thing: the correct hoof-care! Cause of so many maladies!

In the 40 years I have to do with horses, I have seen many different kinds of caring for hooves. As long as hooves and horse are of correct shape and the hoof-care is done regularly and in short enough intervals, there is nearly no difference in the results between most methods. But with deformed hooves and leg-shapes some methods are clearly better than other ones! And the best method I have come up to until now ist the relatively new method called F-Balance, which makes especially use of the high vertical flexibility of the heels of the hoof. The method was tested on racehorses against two other well-known methods by the University of Leipzig and was found superior to them. Because of this I learned the method and now apply it successfully myself! You can read more about this method on the website http://www.f-balance.com/en/ .

I am very confident that the treatments described in this book will also help a lot of horses in English speaking countries!

I wish you every success!

Stefan Brosig
in December 2018

Foreword to the 1st German edition

"Why doing something in a simple way, if you can do it complicated!" This view unfortunately seems to be quite widespread nowadays. Simplicity also is often treated as equivalent to faultiness.

In this book I would like to point out that simple things sometimes are not only good, but sometimes even better than the complicated ones,. You can find here several treatments for horses which are not only equal to the methods of the classical veterinary medicine but in some regards even distinctly better! If one adapts the dosages appropriately, they can even be applied partially to people.

Stefan Brosig
in December 2006

Foreword to the 2nd supplemental and revised German edition

New knowledge and experiences of many users have made reasonable a supplemental and revised edition. Fortunately, the use of ginger, partially also of horseradish, starts to spread, though slowly, among veterinarians. Even at the universities research about herbal remedies like ginger is on the rise, although in this area no gushing font of money is to be expected from pharmaceutical companies.

However, in my opinion the potential of these remedies is still not fully recognized. Many former investigations should thus be repeated on account of the non-linear correlations, described in this book, between dosage, effect and adverse effects. By increasing the dosages up to the limit of good tolerance, I expect from such investigations many new useful treatments for animals and also for people!

„Against every illness a herb has grown!" says a German proverb. At least one should not disregard it thoughtlessly!

Stefan Brosig
in January 2008

Foreword to the 3rd supplemental and revised German edition

The findings of the last years in the feeding of ginger and horseradish to horses has confirmed what had been found previously, and there have not been found many more new uses for these plants. The knowledge that ginger is of great benefit as a remedy for horses is spreading more and more.

Nevertheless it was time to issue a new edition, because there has been in the mean time significant progress in other areas, e.g. a better tolerated "feeding" of ginger to people by means of a double encapsulation. Moreover, licorice has turned out as a promising remedy to relieve horses of some kinds of headshaking! The first investigations also seem to indicate that it is suitable to fight herpesviruses in horses!

Thus with ginger, horseradish, licorice and mosses, four strong remedies are now available to treat in horses effectively inflammations, bacterial infections, headshaking and fungal skin infections. Besides, some of the methods are well applicable to people!

To fight thrush and also as a prevention against it, an externally applied mixture of oregano, easily dissolvable oat flakes and water has turned out as very effective and at the same time mild.

And sand-cracks in hoofs can be repaired simply by covering and gluing the crack by means of fiberglass fabric and a synthetic resin until the crack has completely grown down.

The fact that ginger is very healthy for people has been known for a very long time! Already Shen Nung, the second Yellow Emperor of China, rated ginger exceedingly high for the human health! He divided medicinal plants into three classes: The "servant-herbs" which were toxic and could only be taken in the smallest amounts, the "minister-herbs" which were not poisonous though, but which one nevertheless should take only for a restricted period of time, and the „royal plants", which were allowed to be taken in larger quantities and for an indefinite period of time, and which protected people against illnesses and maintained their vitality. For the Yellow Emperor ginger was one of the most important plants in this "king's class"!

Although I am no „Yellow Emperor", this statement is in my opinion true also for ginger in the feeding to horses!

I wish you every success in the treatments of your four-legged friends!

Stefan Brosig
in January 2010

Foreword to the 4th supplemental and revised German edition

In the three years since the last revision, enough new experience has accumulated to justify a new edition. An important task of this book is also to make clear to horse owners the difference between inhibition of inflammation and pain inhibition and also between inflammation and infection, because many people confuse these terms to the detriment of their horses, but also to their own!

In the meantime, ginger has also received the "knighthood" by the experts: He has been included in the doping list! Probably it is the only recognized doping drug with no harmful side effects, because even after up to 10 years of continuous use in my sensitive English thoroughbred I can not recognize such side effects. This is the advantage of a food!

And its use spreads more and more to other species. Thus, e.g. even a zebra and an old elephant lady with osteoarthritis (daily dosage 250 grams of African ginger) are treated gently with ginger.

The deworming effect described in the first edition was confirmed even after many years of use, without resistance being observed. However, with one exception: tapeworms! Ginger (just as many of the common deworming agents) does not work against them. Therefore, I recommend the so-called selective deworming, which has become common in some countries and in which the type of worms is determined in faeces samples and then one only treats specifically against those found in the sample.

The treatment of idiopathic headshakers with licorice is not yet common, certainly also because more complex accompanying examinations are recommended during the administration. A stronger distribution would be desirable in my opinion, especially since for my own thoroughbred, now in the fifth year of treatment, a steady decline in headshaking was observed from year to year, allowing that the dosage could be reduced every year. Obviously, there is a partial long-term cure of the cause of his headshaking!

Once again, I wish all the best in the treatment of your horses!

Stefan Brosig
in January 2013

The „main actors" in the history of ginger feeding:

Waran (1971 – 2006)
(at the age of 35 years)

Assi (1974 - 2004)
(at the age of 30 years)

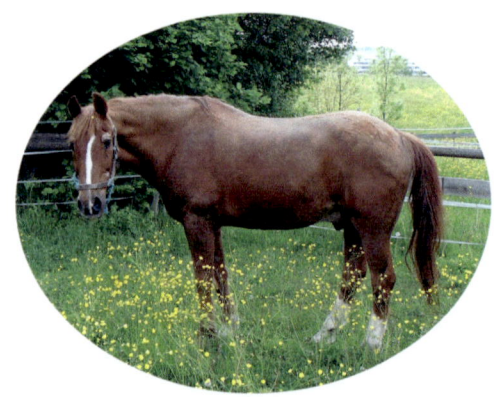

Amarock (*1987)
(at the age of 19 years)

Renaissance Fleur (*1992)
(at the age of 14 years)

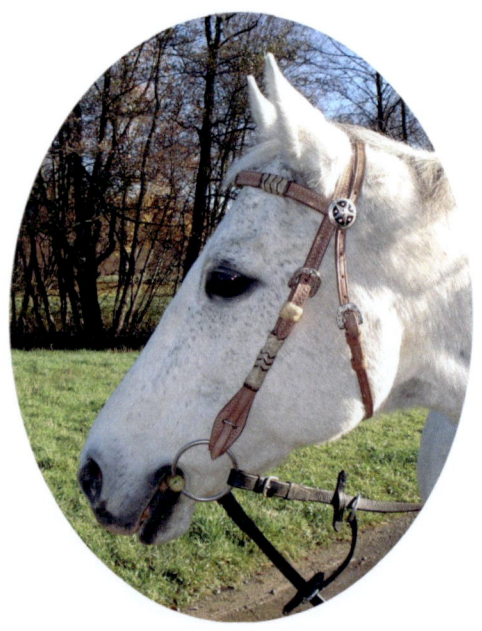
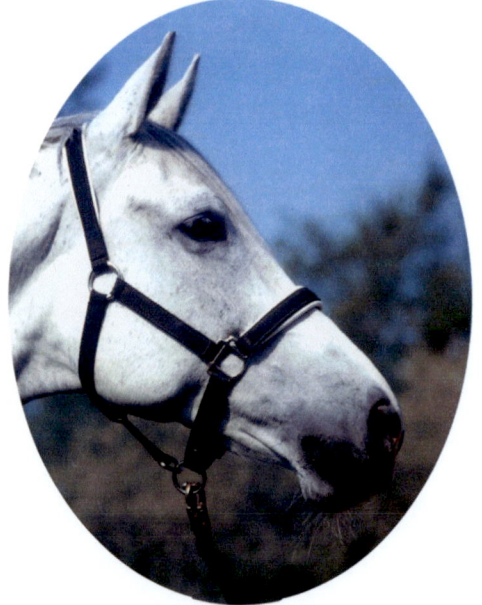

Table of contents

	Introduction	10
A.	Ginger feeding	
	Basics	11
	Historical note	13
	Use	13
	Ginger and doping	30
	Treatment of people and dogs	32
	Use of ginger against other diseases (in humans and animals)	36
	Does ginger have adverse side effects?	48
	Ginger dosages for different diseases of horses (table)	49
	Turmeric as a ginger-substitute?	51
	Frequently asked questions	52
	Quick guide for feeding ginger to horses	60
B.	Horseradish in horse-feeding	62
	Quick guide for feeding horseradish to horses	70
C.	Licorice in horse-feeding	72
	Quick guide for feeding licorice to horses	82
D.	Treatment of fungal skin diseases of horses	83
	Quick guide to treatment of fungal skin infections	85
E.	Ambulant treatment of keratomas	86
F.	Treatment of cracks in hooves (sandcracks)	90
G.	Glued-on dressings	93
H	Gentle method of growth inhibition of equine sarcoids	94

Introduction

Since 2002, **ginger** is used in horses for treatment of a wide range of ailments, especially in cases of injury- or age-related arthrosis and inflammation.

Initially, its use spread only slowly among the horse owners, as ginger was regarded by many physicians and also the pharmaceutical industry with great distrust: In their classical and dogmatic medicinal view a spice had no place within horse medicine. Maybe even worse: it was freely available for everyone and unrivaled cheap.

However, after **Renaissance Fleur** (Trakehner breed), the famous dressage mare and great German hope for the Olympic Games 2004, was treated successfully with ginger since 2003, the use of ginger spread widely among the horse owners.

Targeted examinations or purely random discoveries have added new fields of use beyond the treatment of arthrosis. It turned out that ginger acts „holistically", to use this buzzword for it.

In the meantime, ginger's efficacy, albeit grudgingly, has been recognized, and it has therefore been included in the doping list.

In 2004, **horseradish** has been added to the anti-inflammatory ginger as a broad-band antibiotic, which helps to compensate for this deficiency of ginger.

The use of horseradish (probably also etymologically connected to „horse"), which is superior in some respects even to common pharmaceutical antibiotics, is spreading now too. Also for horseradish there could be the "danger" to be included in the doping list sometime, because he seems to increase the content of young blood pigment (similar to EPO) when fed for several weeks.

In this book, I want to outline the current state of knowledge in the feeding of ginger and horseradish, based on research with my own horses and those of acquaintances, horses of the stud farm Rondeshagen (home of Renaissance Fleur) and on experience reports from many other horse owners (a total of several hundred horses), whom I herewith want to thank a lot for their willingness in giving their reports back to me! Without them, advances in the knowledge would have been significantly slower.

At the end of the book I want to present some other natural products which also deserve to be used on a large scale. With particular emphasis I want to point out the use of **mosses** against fungal skin diseases and of **licorice** (the plant) against pollen-induced headshaking and, eventually, also against herpes infections.

Additionally, you will find a possible ambulant treatment method for **keratomas** in the hoof and a simple method for letting **sandcracks** in the hoof's wall heal and grow down. A caring method for wounds by **glued-on dressings** is also presented. This method I learned from my vet many years ago and it deserves to be saved from oblivion, though vets do not use it any more today, I suppose because they cannot earn something with it. Furthermore, an external treatment of sarcoids alternatingly with liverwort extract and cod liver oil seems to stop or inhibit the growth of equine sarcoids.

A. Ginger

Basics

In horse medicine great progress has been achieved in recent decades, and today it is possible to treat injuries which in earlier times would have been a death sentence. Nevertheless, the medical art of healing still shows some very weak spots that the pharmaceutical industry has not been able to eliminate up to this day.

One of these weak spots is the fight against inflammations and pains without harmful side effects. Up to now available pain-relieving and anti-inflammatory medicines from the group of non-steroidal anti-inflammatory drugs (in short often called NSAIDs or NSARs, non-steroidal anti-inflammatory drugs or non-steroidal antirheumatics) all act aggressively onto the digestive tract after quite a short time. Thus their use must occur over a limited time only and a continuous use in high enough dosage is excluded in case of chronic inflammations and pains, which is so frequent in old age. (Best known to the horse owners is the active substance phenylbutazon, which, for example, is known as Equipalazone®).

Another weak spot is "The lost art of healing" itself, as the American physician and Nobel Prize Laureate Bernard Lown complains about in his book with the same title. Medicine has become more and more of an emergency medicine.

In aftercare and long-term healing of a disease, people, as well as horse owners, are often left alone to themselves.

But Australian scientists of the Herbal Medicine Research and Education Centre and the University of Queensland helped out with a discovery from Mother Nature to remove these weak spots in many cases:

In 2001 they found that the spice ginger, or an essence from it, reduces the sensation of pain in rats and has an anti-inflammatory effect!

Ginger is the root (more precisely, the rhizome) of the reed-like ginger shrub (Zingiber officinale) which is cultivated from India to China, in other tropical areas and also in Africa, and is traded as a spice fresh or dried. Most people will know ginger as a powder from the spice rack in the super market.

Ginger does not act homeopathically or like a placebo, but according to conventional medicine: Certain compounds in ginger, above all probably the so-called gingerols and shogaols, the essential pungent ingredients of ginger, dock at the same (so-called "vanilloid") receptors in the cells as for example the non-steroidal anti-inflammatory drugs Ibuprofen®, Aspirin® and also Equipalazone®. However, ginger does not show the serious side effects which are connected with the intake of the usual non-steroidal anti-inflammatory drugs! For ginger no contraindications are known in people. Even pregnant women may take it for a long time against nausea (Obstetrics & Gynecology, Vol. 105, April, 2005).

Surprisingly, in relation to body weight, ginger acts significantly more pain-relieving and anti-inflammatory in horses than in rats.

Experiences have also shown that ginger is first and foremost an anti-inflammatory drug and that it effectively eliminates pain especially, when the pain is due to an inflammation!

Historical note

The horse which was the first to receive ginger daily in larger amounts and in long term as a feed supplement was my warmblood gelding Waran (born in 1971, died in July 2006, as a consequence of a completely toothless lower jaw). To treat a strong inflammation of his hoof-joint he had received ginger (in dry, ground form) starting in March 2002 over a period of more than 7 months in a pain-relieving and anti-inflammatory amount of about 3 grams per 100 kilograms of body weight, and thereafter he received it further in amounts which varied experimentally between 1.5 and 4 grams per 100 kilograms of body weight, because it obviously was good for him. In the last 2 years of his life he received daily amounts of 3 to 4 grams per 100 kilograms of body weight without any sign of adverse effects.
Hence, a picture (at the age of 35 years) of my very affectionate gelding, whom I will never forget, decorates the back-cover of this book.

Since my letters to editors of horse magazines, ginger has already saved the life of many other horses and made life easier for even more! It is already used by studs as a kind of routine treatment, independent of race, be it Icelandic, Trakehner or thoroughbred.
The most prominent "ginger eater" and at the same time "blockade runner" against the prejudice of many veterinarians at that time that ginger would act only like a placebo, is probably the Trakehner mare Renaissance Fleur, who tragically suffered a triple debris fracture of her fetlock and its joint in February 2003 while in a training stable. (This accident also shattered the hope of this best German dressage mare for a medal at the Olympic Games 2004.) The leg was set together in an emergency operation with nine (!) screws like a mosaic. The horse's weight was simultaneously transferred to the hoof via an outer cast around the fetlock. A proof of what can be done now by modern medical science! However, when the mare left the clinic after four months, she was getting worse from day to day. The fetlock joint stiffened (deliberately) completely. Finally, the mare was completely lame because of strong arthrosis and lost more and more weight. (At that time most horse magazines reported about this).

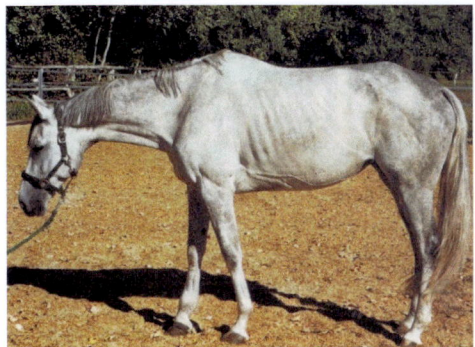 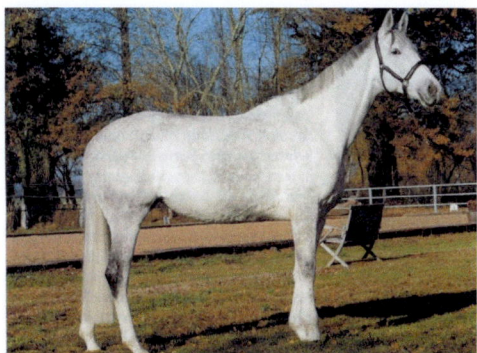

The left picture shows Renaissance Fleur in August 2003, after her return to the stud; the right picture shows her in November after only 2 months of feeding ginger.

By feeding of ginger a painless walking and also trotting was again possible for the mare since September 2003. This made the way free for a hopefully long and trouble-free life of this great mare. The mare felt increasingly better under ginger, and she could also gallop again across the pasture, despite her stiff fetlock joint. The affected leg also became a bit thinner again over time. So nothing prevented her use as a content brood mare. In April 2006, Renaissance Fleur got her first filly, Roulette, fit as a fiddle. Then in 2008 there came the second filly, Reminescence, and in 2010 the third healthy foal, again a filly, Residence. In 2011 she had a twin birth, of which unfortunately neither of the two foals was viable. The birth had been a great emotional burden, but the mare quickly recovered by the good care.

The picture on the front cover shows her in 2006 together with her first filly, her mother Regatta (died in October, 2009 at the age of 29 ½ years) and her owner and breeder in the stud Rondeshagen.

Since the beginning of 2003 a study was running by the Reha team Aggertal (head M. Hompesch) in which ginger is applied highly dosed and successfully to horses who could not been helped by conventional veterinary treatment anymore and were resistant to therapy. These horses suffer from extreme arthrosis in several joints simultaneously, high-grade spavin on both sides, high-grade podotrochlosis (navicular disease), high-grade ataxia or Wobbler-syndrome (cervical vertebral malformation, CVM), calcifications and other diseases.

Although a treatment with ginger is a little bit more time-consuming and the effect appears only with a bit greater delay than with medicines which are used by vets to treat inflammations and pains, the **advantages** of ginger prevail by far:
- **no adverse side effects**
- **no contraindications and**
- **no waiting periods**,
because ginger is a food.
Besides, it is inexpensive.
Veterinarians may have faster acting remedies in their funds, but none that are better and healthier!
Hence, ginger is to be looked upon as the means of choice and should always be used, at least if a long-term use of an anti-inflammatory substance is necessary. Actually one follows only one motto of the ancient Hippokrates (about 460-375 B.C.): „Let food be your remedy, and remedy be your food!"

Use

For the horse owner, practical instructions for use are particularly interesting, because he himself is required to determine the individually required dosage for his horse. In the following I would like to enumerate the essential points that have to be considered for a successful treatment of the horse:

1.) Ginger is a **natural product**, and its pain-relieving and anti-inflammatory effect is highly dependent on its origin and its content of active ingredients. These are mainly the **pungent substances**, especially the **gingerols**, which in customary dry ginger powder range between 0.5 and 3%. Ginger from Africa (Tanzania, Nigeria), usually has the highest content of gingerols, but there are also very good qualities from other countries (sometimes with certificated content of pungent substances of about 2% or more). Today one can buy ginger of good quality via internet, at least in Germany. In Germany also many of the big horseware-traders deal with it now (e.g. Masterhorse). However, there are also "black sheep" who sell bad Asian qualities as good ginger! (When comparing different ginger qualities one should also consider the kind of the used analysis! The more simple photometric determinations show distinctly higher contents than those which use HPLC (high pressure liquid chromatography) with which the material mixture to be analysed is separated into its components before analysis! HPLC seems indeed to show values which are very slightly below the true content.)

As an up-to now experience, ginger from Africa has shown to be always equivalent to ginger from other areas of the world, even if its content of pungent substances was only about 1.5%. (Such ginger is e.g. better accepted by picky "gourmet horses"!) An explanation for this may be that African ginger, even if of lower content in anti-inflammatory substances, at the same time contains a lower concentration in pro-inflammatory substances and that it is the difference between both classes of substances which is decisive for the overall effect. Besides, further active substances seem to be involved in the anti-inflammatory and analgesic effect of ginger! (One such substance which is included in African ginger in clearly higher amounts than in Asian ginger is, e.g., zingiberene. (For this, see the dissertation of A. Riyazi, Univ. Münster, Pharmakologische Untersuchungen zum antiemetischen Wirkungsmechanismus des ätherischen Öls von Ingwer (Zingiber officinale Roscoe)). For example, ginger has also proved effective for treatment of horses which were indifferent to treatment with phenylbutazone, an NSAID. This shows that (at least) one other additional active mechanism must exist for which other substances than the gingerols must be responsible. Grzanna et al. describe such an additional mechanism in J. Med. Food, 2005, 8 (2), pp. 125-132: on the one hand ginger suppresses the synthesis of the pro-inflammatory prostaglandin by inhibiting the enzymes cyclooxygenase-1 and cyclooxygenase-2 (COX-1 and COX -2). But unlike "chemical" non-steroidal anti-inflammatory drugs it additionally suppresses the formation of pro-inflammatory leukotriene by inhibiting the 5-lipoxygenase!

The ground ginger from the supermarket is more expensive and older than that from the special traders and, unfortunately, it is also not specified in its content of pungent substances or its origin. Although one can find good qualities there too, often however, you will find also bad or even very bad qualities, which hardly work or even not at all. In most cases these are Asian grades with a low content of pungent substances.

However, ginger powder from the supermarket is definitely sufficient to get a horse used to the taste, so that in case of emergency later on there will be no acceptance problems.

In old, poorly stored ginger the gingerols have often converted partly into **zingerone**. Hence, a high content of zingerone is a criterion for a poorer quality of ginger. Even if old ginger with high a content of zingerone is not very suitable for the treatment of inflammations, it may have merit in the treatment of some kinds of **diarrhea**; the reason is, that it is just the content of zingerone that is important for the good effect against such diarrheas (J. Agric. Food Chem., 2007, 55, (21), p. 8390-8397).

With **fresh ginger** you pay primarily the water (about 85%), and mostly these are Asian sorts with a low content of pungent substances. In terms of effectiveness, however, the **fresh state** seems to **compensate** in part for the lower level of sharpness. Ginger powder from the chemist's shop usually is more expensive and often also noticeably worse, because the gingerols are slowly converted during storage into so-called (and even more pungent) **shogaols** which are less effective. Hence, preferentially larger amounts of ginger are best to be stored in closed vessels in the fridge, and the amount for at most two months may be bottled in a smaller tight-fitting vessel at room temperature for direct use. **(When in this book the word "ginger" is used, the dried form is meant in general.)**

(By the way, the pungent substance of **chili** and cayenne pepper, **capsaicin**, is also pain-relieving and anti-inflammatory. However, in contrast to the pungent ingredients of ginger, in the high amounts necessary for inhibition of pain and inflammation it acts destructive on mucous membranes!)

2.) With horses who are treated with ginger f**or the first time**, it is necessary to **increase the amount slowly**. As experience shows, especially highly-bred animals can be picky in this respect. Also horses in stables, in which they have always free access to feed and thus are always saturated, can show greater restraints against ginger.

Thus it is best to begin with very small amounts of ginger; usually a total quantity of about 1 gram in the principal meal is well accepted by most horses. The next day one can usually increase to 3 grams, then to 6 grams and then further on in steps of 3 grams.

With **sensitive horses**, which react to changes of feed with health difficulties (e.g. colics), this should happen **more slowly** than with standard ones, for which only several days are needed to increase the amount to the necessary final dosage.

For horses with severe **renal insufficiency** one must take into account that the active substances of ginger are eliminated from the body substantially slower. The dosage in these cases should in some cases be significantly reduced and the increasing of the amount from day to day should occur more slowly.

Preferably, ginger is offered in soaked (however, not dripping, but "earth-humid") **hay-/grasscubes** of good quality (rich in fiber). Ginger thereby becomes substantially more acceptable for the horse because its smell and sharpness are significantly reduced. In soaked hay-/grasscubes one can feed to horses triple to four-fold the amount of ginger as compared to feeding in rolled oats. In soaked hay-/grasscubes it is thus possible to feed large amounts of ginger in one serving. An amount of **20 to 30 grams of ginger** can be served to the horse, well accepted, in about **half a kilogram (dry matter) of hay-/grasscubes** plus the amount of water necessary for soaking.

If you use **shredded hay-/grasscubes** (often supplied for old horses), the time of soaking shortens considerably. In a shredded state, the quantity of water necessary for soaking, can be measured more exactly, so that the feed is only "humid", and not „sappily dripping", because many horses do not like this. This may be because the taste of ginger is then not hidden in the fiber, but is also partially present in the free liquid and thus tastes stronger.

One can also add **boiled linseeds, bananas, fine cut carrots or apples**, especially at the beginning when the ginger is still unknown to the horse. The rehab team Aggertal makes their high dosages tasty to the horses by means of **citrus fruits**. Others use brewer's yeast to mask the smell, or some drops of peppermint oil.

I myself have made good experiences with adding **previously boiled linseed** (about 50 grams), one mashed **banana**, and 30 milliliter of **black caraway oil** to mask about 40 grams of ginger in 600 grams of hay-/grasscubes plus water.

Very easy is also the use of fructose. Unlike normal sugar or glucose, fructose has the property of not increasing insulin levels! Up to amounts of about 100 grams per day, the administration of fructose in the horse is to be regarded as uncritical. This amount is e.g. already contained in about a kilogram of sweet apples. With one to two grams of fructose per gram of ginger, one can "sweeten" the ginger for a picky horse. Even with horses that do not like soaked hay-/grasscubes it makes sense to make them tasty with fructose, because giving ginger in soaked hay-/grasscubes has so many advantages that one should try many things to make them tasty! Once they have found a liking for them, one can usually leave the fructose away or reduce it by and by.

A particularly advantageous way to supply the required ginger amount to "gourmet" horses is the use of ginger in a **coarser state** which smells and tastes less strongly. The very coarse cut form (looks like dried mushrooms) is generally accepted well, however, it is also utilized less completely, depending on the degree of chewing. Part of it just comes out "backwards". It can happen then that one must feed double the amount compared to ground ginger, sometimes even more.

A preferable state is granulated or fine cut. (I myself like to use the granulated Nigerian ginger from the company Masterhorse.)

Another possibility for getting the horse accustomed to ginger is feeding it as fresh ginger, which is liked by many horses. But because this contains a lot of water, this must be accounted for and a substantially larger amount is required compared to the dried product!

Owners of extreme "gourmet" horses have successfully mixed the ginger powder with a vegetable oil (many use oil of sunflower seeds, I myself prefer oil of thistle seeds), applesauce or fruit juice, and then infused the mixture **directly into the mouth** of their horses **with a big syringe**. (Oil may be advantageous, because fats in general "bind" sharpness.) After some time the horses get used to it, and when they have realized that ginger is doing them good, they often accept it directly in their food. Maybe this is the method of choice, if there is no time to accustom picky horses by slow, patient raising of the amount of ginger. But here too one must not immediately administer the final high dosage immediately on the first day but increase it slowly (as should be done with every horse feed).

Other methods found by creative horse owners, can be found in the chapter "**Frequently asked questions**".

Presumably it is primarily the **smell** and less the sharpness which **irritates** the horses most. (Hence, a ginger with a lower content of the smell-causing essential oils is advantageous for "gourmet" horses, at least in the beginning.) In general, horses seem to have little sense of taste for sharpness. (This is also evident, e.g., from the fact that they eat horseradish and garlic.) After they notice that ginger helps them, some horses are even downright "sharp" to eat it, and, incredibly, some eat ginger powder even in pure state!

In **later treatments**, when the horse already knows ginger, the dosage can be increased **very quickly**. It is then usually possible to start immediately with the standard dosage of 3 to 4 grams per 100 kilograms of body weight and increase this dosage quickly further if necessary (for example in case of inflammations of "soft parts", e.g. tendons or ligaments).

And in horses, which already permanently receive a "joint dosage" of 3 to 4 grams per 100 kilograms of body weight, you can usually, for example in case of a soft tissue inflammation, immediately increase the required dosage to 10 to 15 grams per 100 kilograms of body weight.

For this reason it makes sense to **get horses used to the taste of ginger early**, even if they do not need it at that time at all. Because then, if necessary, there will be no problems of acceptance, and one can increase the dosage fast to the necessary amount.

For the same reason it also makes sense to **get horses already used to soaked hay-/grass cubes**, because some horses might not like them at the beginning.

However, they make the feeding of ginger so much easier that this time and effort are worthwhile later on. When the horses have learned to appreciate the cubes, one can quit feeding them again until a case of illness arises which makes the feeding of ginger necessary.

By the way, hay-/grasscubes are also valuable for "hiding" other medicines for horses!

Some horses prefer alfalfa-cubes to hay-/grasscubes. But it is important to ensure that the amount is not too large, because alfalfa is very rich in calcium! An excessively high ratio of calcium to phosphorus in the feed can increase the bony deposits (exostoses), especially in horses with osteoarthritis! For the same reason, it must be warned from the addition of calcium supplements, if there is no calcium deficiency! Such a deficiency must be previously proven, otherwise calcium does harm and leads to deposits in the joints and tendons (particularly in combination with excess vitamin D!).

But in the case of bone-degrading spavin, alfalfa is advantageous.

Also in horses with weak bones alfalfa in an amount of up to 1 kilogram per day is not questionable. On the other hand, horses with exostoses by arthrosis should stay well below that.

Freshly built up bony structures within the joint space and in soft tissues seem to be diminished or even completely eliminated again by ginger over time, as also Hekla Lava seems to do. But there is no influence of ginger on the size of old exostoses.

3.) For **diseases** which concern **only the joints**, the daily dosage at which a strong pain-relieving and anti-inflammatory effect is observable with most horses, is **about 3 grams (dry grade) per 100 kilograms of body weight** when using African ginger or a ginger quality containing about 2% of pungent substances or more.

As with people, the **dosage** can also be **individually different**, that is lower or higher. Nevertheless, 15 grams daily for a horse weighing 500 kilograms are a very good reference value. (Today, however, many warmblood horses weigh clearly more than 500 kilograms!)

Once you have reached the estimated dosage for the horse in question, you can wait two more days before a further increase of the amount, because it is a characteristic of the treatment with ginger that it **starts to show an effect**, virtually all of a sudden, **about one and a half to two days after reaching the necessary dosage which is individual for the horse and the kind of illness**. And this effect usually further increases a bit during the following days ******. (The reason for this delayed effect is probably that **ginger is primarily anti-inflammatory**. An observable inhibition of pain is distinctly noticeable only when the cause of the pain, namely the inflammation, has been significantly suppressed.)

If there is still **no recognizable effect at the dosage estimated for the respective horse**, the amount of ginger must be **increased further**. (It is favorable for a horse of about 500 kilograms of body weight to heighten the daily amount in 3-gram increments. With higher necessary dosages, 5-gram steps or even more make sense). Observations have shown that a dosage of about **3 grams per 100 kilograms of body weight has to be exceeded** (by about a factor ranging from 3 to 4) if, besides the joints, also **"soft parts" (e. g. tendons, ligaments, muscles) are affected** to a greater extent.

Should the required amount for a distinct reduction of lameness be substantially higher than 3 grams per 100 kilograms of body weight, this is an indication that the diagnosis "joints" is not complete. Hence, ginger could be used by the veterinarian as a **diagnostic aid** to distinguish between both cases.

The **maximum total amounts of ginger** known to me to have been necessary for a horse per day **over a long term** amounted to **160 grams** (about 30 grams per 100 kilograms of body weight!) and were given for 8 to 9 months (carried out by the rehab team Aggertal)! For a little borreliosis-afflicted Shetland pony, suffering simultaneously from laminitis (founder) and metabolic syndrome, amounts of more than 60 grams per 100 kilograms of body weight were necessary and given by a private horse owner to improve the lameness noticeably. (For a short time even up to 120 grams per 100 kilograms of body weight were given, and, easily comprehensible, with huge problems of acceptance!) However, with these huge dosages long-term experience is missing! I myself have already fed 40 grams of ginger (coarsely cut) per 100 kilograms of body weight for more than two months to my old warmblood gelding Waran because of a partly ruptured muscle. For his weight this was an everyday total quantity of about 200 grams.

For every horse, for which the usual non-steroidal anti-inflammatory drugs are effective, ginger will also act beneficially, because the mechanism of inhibition of inflammation is in part identical. However, in addition, ginger has also turned out to be effective for horses who did not respond to phenylbutazone any more. This demonstrates that ginger, composed of many components, does also act by **additional other mechanisms**.

(Regarding the **pain inhibition independent of the inflammation inhibition**, however, **phenylbutazone** is stronger than ginger. In exchange, the anti-inflammatory potential of ginger excels that of phenylbutazone, because as foodstuff ginger can be dosed almost arbitrarily high (up to the limit of acceptance).)

Having once determined the necessary daily minimum dosage for the horse in question, it makes sense to **heighten** this further **as a safety margin** by about 20% to compensate for inaccuracies of dosage and variations in sensitivities from day to day. For total quantities up to about 100 grams per day, and when feeding in soaked hay-/grasscubes, it is not necessary to divide the dosage into two meals per day (except in case of problems of acceptance). With **higher amounts** a **split into several servings** is advantageous. (E.g., after getting used to ginger, 20 grams of ginger, or even more, can be "hidden" with good acceptance in about 500 grams (dry matter) of soaked hay-/grasscubes. In a coarser form, even distinctly more ginger can be "hidden" in the hay-/grasscubes.) By the way, if you allow **soaking of ginger and hay-/grass-cubes together**, it is accepted **even better**.

Cool weather supports the treatment of inflammations with ginger: in hot weather a higher dosage is usually necessary than in "November weather".

Warm **wrapping up of the joints** of horses with arthrosis in winter is in my opinion not necessary when feeding ginger, maybe even bad, since long-term wrapping usually is not beneficial for legs. However, this certainly varies individually from animal to animal!

** Instead of pausing at the initially estimated necessary amount of ginger for about 2 days before increasing the amount again, you can also, on account of the harmlessness of ginger which has proved itself now over many years, increase the amount further on, until a distinct positive effect shows. Although you have then crossed the necessary threshold amount for the corresponding horse and illness a bit, this does not matter! The horse is painless earlier, and you can lower the ginger amount later still, if you like to do so! Therefore, this is even the preferential approach in many cases and has thus become the standard procedure for me! However, with risk horses, e.g. those tending to colics or with renal insufficiency, one has to proceed more careful!

4.) During the first month of treatment, the horse may (but need not) get less sensitive to ginger, as it is also the case with all pain-relieving and anti-inflammatory medicines. This may require an increase of the dosage once again by about 20%. In the following years, however, this dosage remains constant according to past experience (even for years).
Since ginger has proved to be harmless even when feeding it for a very long time (more than 10 years), I have now since some time even begun to exceed the required threshold amount by about 50%, although it would actually not be necessary. However, it has a possible additional benefit if there should, for example, be present undiagnosed soft tissue inflammations, or a tumor, the growth of which would then be slowed down at least a bit.

5.) As already mentioned, the **sharp transition** from an unobservable effect to a distinct effect, which can be observed with an only slight increase of the ginger amount, is remarkable. (This can be observed in particular with mere joint diseases, with soft tissue inflammations this threshold is less sharp). This transition takes place in a rather narrow range of only about 20% of the total necessary dosage. It may be that with 12 grams per day there is still no effect recognizable and with 15 grams the horse suddenly bucks with joy and trots away across the pasture, as, for example, it had been the case with Renaissance Fleur.
Slightly below the threshold amount at which pain-relieving and anti-inflammatory effects can suddenly be observed, sometimes an **increase in pain** can happen. Hence, this line should be crossed fast! (To avoid unnecessary suffering of the horse, it makes sense not to play around for too long whether 3 grams per 100 kilos of body weight are sufficient for a treatment or not, but to increase the dosage quickly until a significant improvement in the horse can be observed. Then later on, one can still try to reduce this dosage again.)
This case is schematically shown in the following figure which represents the relative sensation of joint pain at a given dosage of ginger:

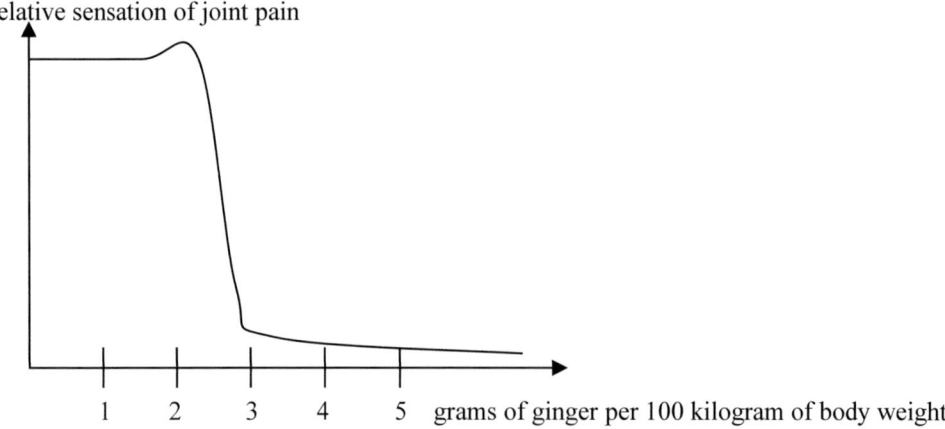

relative sensation of joint pain

1 2 3 4 5 grams of ginger per 100 kilogram of body weight

The reason for this sharp threshold certainly is, that ginger contains hundreds of active substances which influence themselves mutually, whereas traditional drugs are mostly pure substances or contain only very few other substances.

Therefore, the anti-inflammatory properties of gingerols (and other ingredients) seem to be down-regulated first by other ingredients with opposite effect (antagonists) when using only low sub-threshold ginger amounts, and then to rise almost all of a sudden on account of a **non-linear behavior** when concentrations in the body increase beyond a certain concentration.

The use of counteracting means to create such **steep characteristic curves** (non-linear relation between cause (here: dosage of ginger) and effect (here: feeling of pain)) is well-known in many areas of engineering and science (e.g.: transistor). But today's medicine with its treatment of substantially more complicated systems is still a long way from that.

Hence, the effects of ginger described in this book have so far been simply overlooked because the necessary high dosages were simply never tested: the strong observed effects cannot be deduced from the action behavior at low dosages by simple linear extrapolation!

Since such **pairing of agonists/antagonists** is a **principle which is common in nature**, this means that for some other natural substances, too, afore misjudged or unrecognized effects can be expected after crossing a certain threshold because of such non-linear behavior!

Apparently **horseradish** also is such a natural substance with extraordinary effects (in this case highly antibiotic)! You will find more exact instructions for its use in **part B** of this book.

Also the combination of ingredients in the (not completely uncritical) plant **licorice** shows remarkable effects in horses, and these are therefore written down in **part C** of this book.

6.) Ginger is given in the necessary amount, until the inflammation has healed. (For hoof joint inflammations this can be several weeks or many months, depending on the severity of the special case!) Then the daily amount is lowered again continuously. It goes without saying that until complete healing is reached, the painlessness may not be exploited for usual work of the horse, because otherwise the cause of the suppressed inflammation can worsen!

In the treatment of **soft tissue inflammations** (ligaments, tendons), which sometimes occur (unrecognized) simultaneously to the joint disease and become apparent by the relatively high necessary dosages of ginger (**about 10 to 12 grams per 100 kilograms of body weight**, some horses needing more, some less), it makes sense to maintain this high dosage at first for 4 weeks and then try to lower to a usual "joint dosage" of 3 to 4 grams per 100 kilograms of body weight (best when the weather turns cooler). This dosage should then be maintained for several months until complete healing has taken place. After that a "well-being dosage" of 1.5 to 2 grams per 100 kilograms of body weight should be given for some months further on to support healing of unrecognized very small damages.

The **time for a lowering of the amount** of ginger has come in the majority of cases, when the sick body part is no longer warmer than the same healthy body part on the other side of the horse.

For safety's sake, less experienced horse owners should rely on the judgment of an experienced vet!

My own experiences show that with horses, which had a strong inflammation, it makes sense to give them ginger permanently in a "well-being dosage" of 1.5 to 2 grams per 100 kilo of body weight, since such former sites of inflammation not seldom remain weak spots in which inflammations will flare up again more easily. Because the experiences of the past 11 years, since feeding ginger first started in 2002, have shown that also the "joint dosage" of 3 to 4 grams per 100 kilograms of body weight will in the long term show no adverse side effects, it even makes sense to feed permanently this "joint dosage", because by doing so, freshly emerging inflammations are already stifled at the very beginning. However, this requires a great deal of experience by the horse owner in what horses may be expected to do at work without overloading them!

There is still a further advantage if you continue to feed at least the "well-being dosage" of ginger after the healing of an inflammation: ginger is **accelerating healing processes**, and it also causes **reduction of connective tissue** ("knobs") which has remained at the previously diseased site. This effect usually becomes observable about 6 to 8 weeks after the healing of the inflammation.

As a newer example, my English thoroughbred (22-year-old at the time of the injury) had kicked out unfortunately with his hind legs at a stationary wooden bench for pedestrians on 28 July 2009 and thereby injured his right hind leg. The pictures describe the course of the healing and at the same time also demonstrate the use of horseradish and glued-on dressings, described in more detail in later chapters:

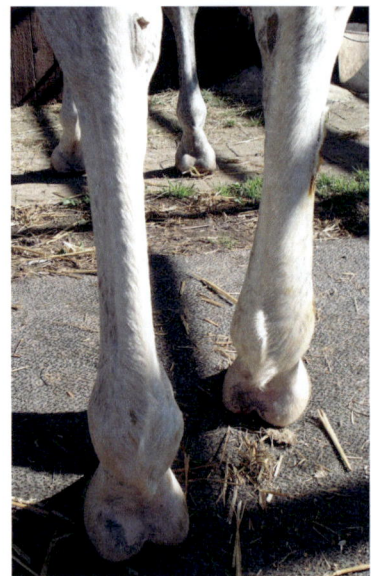 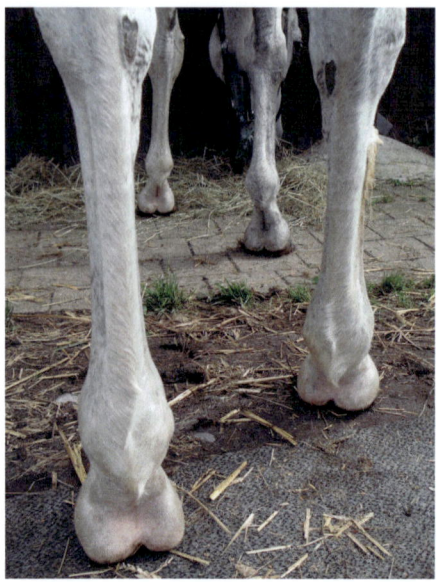

On July 29th the right hind leg had swollen on account of the skin injury (already cared for on the day before with a glued-on dressing) to a small to medium sized phlegmon.
From this day on the horse received 25 grams of horseradish per 100 kilograms of body weight and 5 grams of ginger per 100 kilograms of body weight.

On August 3rd the phlegmon was completely gone by the antibiotic effect of highly-dosed horseradish. Most of the swelling had already disappeared on July 30th. However, small movable knobs remained at the place of the hit after recession of the swelling. The glued-on dressing which stuck to the leg all the time, can still be seen.

The white horse had since 2003 been receiving ginger for 6 years at a dosage of about 4 grams (since 2010 about 5 grams) per 100 kilograms of body weight to prevent the enlargement of small melanomas at the underside of the tail. Longtime experience has shown that without ginger the phlegmon would have clearly been bigger from the beginning, because ginger alone reduces swellings of this kind a bit on account of its anti-inflammatory and slightly diuretic properties.
At the beginning of 2010 the knobs were not visible anymore and only could be sensed by someone who knew exactly where to feel.

As it lasts from one and a half to two days, until the therapeutically effective amounts of active substances have accumulated in the body, it also lasts a comparable time, until they have been excreted again! This has the big advantage for the horse owner that with a **one-time daily feeding** of ginger quite a uniform effect can be achieved in the body. **For a quite complete excretion of the active substances of ginger out of the body one should stop feeding it about 5 to 7 days earlier.**

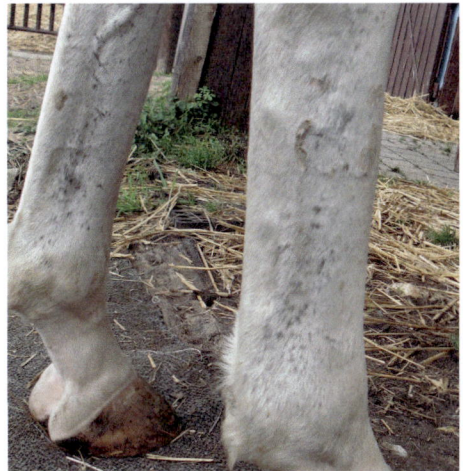
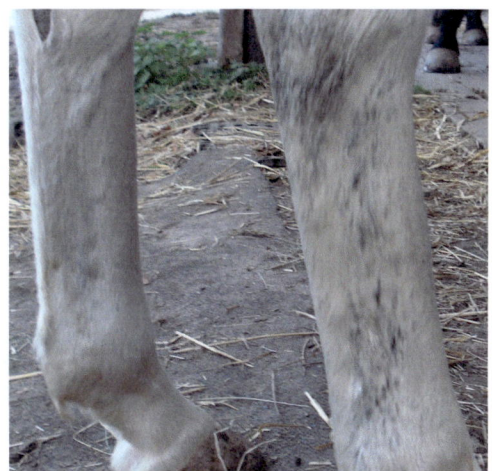

On August 21st the firm knobs shown here have remained. The ginger dosage had already been reduced for 2 weeks to 4 grams per 100 kilograms of body weight again, a dosage which the horse already has been receiving for 6 years as a long-term dosage against his melanomas.

On November 28th the knobs on the leg are already significantly reduced. The beginning of a distinct decline was noticeable from the beginning of October. (The leg has been wetted with water because of the winter coat to make the remains of the knobs more visible.)

7.) For **old horses** a permanent administration of about half of the threshold amount until the end of life seems to be of advantage (**"well-being dosage"**, that is 1.5 to 2 grams per 100 kilograms of body weight). (For horse owners who are already well versed with horses and can well estimate the tolerable work dependent on age (!), even a higher permanent dosage of 3 to 4 grams per 100 kilograms of body weight is recommendable because this dosage shows some additional advantages as compared to the lower dosage!)

I would advise this **from an age of about 12 to 15 years**, even if there are still no, even minor, ailments perceptible. By this the blood becomes a little bit more fluid (however, not much), healings also take place faster in the extremities which are less supplied with blood (see previous pictures). Thromboses disappear in time or get smaller, legs get less edemas, the heart gets less stressed, the change of coat seems to happen faster. The horses are getting "younger" again.

A series of blood tests in recent years on my English thoroughbred at the age of 22 to 25 years and on a Trakehner gelding aged 18 to 19 years indicate very strongly that the amount of the "stress hormone" cortisol in the blood is reduced significantly by ginger! It was below the average value of middle-aged horses and was like that of a young horse! The reductions to about 2 µg / dl were significant with both horses (normal range 2.9 to 9.1 µg / dl in middle-aged horses)! This observation, even if at the time of printing of this book only directly measured in two horses (cortisol is no standard value in blood testing), would be a good explanation for the fact that ginger helps horses with **Cushing syndrome**, because in equine Cushing syndrome the production of cortisol is heightened! Usually this is found especially in older horses. Ginger seems to reduce this excessive production of cortisol considerably or accelerates its decomposition, in horses without Cushing syndrome even below the normal levels of horses of middle or higher age.

However, this does by no means harm to the horses! The levels are just like in young horses again! The anti-inflammatory effects of cortisol are apparently partially taken over by the herbal anti-inflammatory substances of ginger, and this causes the body to produce less cortisol. The reports to the effect of ginger on Equine Cushing which I have received up to now suggest a dosage of about 3 to 4 grams per 100 kilograms of body weight as a guideline for a treatment, in severe cases more.

The lowering of the cortisol level in the blood could also be an explanation for the fact that even old "ginger horses" change their winter coat more easily.

By how much ginger increases the **life expectancy** of horses cannot be told exactly yet, and it is of course dependent on the work load. But I estimate the increase for horses kept in charity to **at least 1 to 2 years**! (By additional feeding of **horseradish** in intervals it can be increased even further! See part B of this book!)

This is related to the effects of ginger observed in humans due to the totality of its ingredients:

Inhibition of aggregation of platelets in the blood, vasodilator effect, increase of the metabolism, digestive, presumably anti-carcinogenic. (According to my own investigations this is certain at least for some kinds of cancer!)

8.) I strongly advise against a long-lasting feeding of commercially available **ginger extracts**! The pure gingerols, like all non-steroidal anti-inflammatory drugs (NSAIDs), irritate the digestive tract! It is the content of many further ingredients in the whole plant of ginger which is responsible for the pronounced **digestibility** of the whole plant. Thus, for example, the present "record" for feeding of sharp dry ginger powder to a Shetland pony with borreliosis, laminitis and metabolic syndrome is 65 grams per 100 kilograms of body weight for at least one month (short-termed even 120 grams per 100 kilograms of body weight), and this even together with 50 grams of horseradish per 100 kilograms of body weight!

However, these are quantities which I would not like to recommend as a standard; these are amounts which one should only test in cases of absolute emergency and accompanied by a vet!

(I myself have already fed 40 grams per 100 kilograms of body weight for more than 2 months, with short-term peaks of up to 65 grams per 100 kilograms of body weight. Very large amounts of ginger should always be given in coarser form (e.g. fine cut or similar) and in quite large quantities of hay-/grasscubes and be distributed among several meals a day!)

9.) All kinds of influences which can negatively affect inflammations in the body should be avoided as far as possible. These are for example too much and wrong work loads and **feed which is unsuitable** for horses. Also people with joint diseases will receive a "diet" and not just "normal" food.

Feed stuff for which there exists a danger of an increase of inflammations can be found in feeds to which horses are not adapted to in the course of evolution. According to my observations especially **bread** can intensify already existing inflammations. The reason might lie in the flavoring substances formed by heating. However, also **easily digestible carbohydrates** might be responsible. This would mean that sugar and also grass rich in fructans could be harmful in this respect. Insulin levels thus increased are also linked to inflammations in people (e.g. even in the brain: Fishel, archive of Neurology, Vol. 62, p. 1, 2005). Although in healthy horses no obvious influence on the joints is evident, I believe that bread should better be eliminated completely from the diet of horses. Incidentally, old horse people have always warned against bread as horse feed.

10.) Long-term feeding of ginger in a dosage of already 1.5 to 2 grams per 100 kilograms of body weight and day (warmbloods) leads to **elimination** or **very clear reduction of worm infestation** in many horses!

For dogs and sheep there already exist clinical studies for these results (Iqbal et.al., J. Ethnopharmacol., 2006, 106, p. 285 ff).

For people too it is known that **spices can suppress parasitic infestations**. It is also known, that ginger is traditionally used in tropical countries against bilharziosis (schistosomiasis), which is also caused by worms.

After 3 weeks, in case of strong infestations after about 6 weeks, the animals are **"free" of worms**, if the pastures are not too strongly infested with worm eggs.

However, I have also got knowledge of cases in which ginger could not remove the worms (but such cases also exist with conventional dewormings), hence, the success should be controlled after this period by a fecal test. However, the anti-worm effect is usually already observable by weight gain and a shiny coat.

On the other hand, tapeworms seem to be excluded from the vermifuge action of ginger! These worms must be specifically eliminated with a specific agent (for example, praziquantel) if suspected!

African ginger with a content of pungent ingredients of approximately 1.5% and less than 2% of essential oils also has this deworming effect. I suspect that a variety of substances are responsible for the worming effect, and not just pungent substances and/or essential oils.

So far all horses, which I am personally acquainted with and which are treated with ginger for at least 6 weeks, were "free" of worms afterwards. However, all these animals were fed on completely or nearly completely natural feed. The cases known to me, in which ginger had not been sufficient, had all received feed fortified with supplements and/or supplements directly. Hence, I suspect that in genetically predestined animals some of the supplements in these feeds promote the development of worms so strongly that the gently deworming effect of ginger cannot compensate the worm-nurturing action of these supplements. Which of these supplements could be responsible for it, I do not know. A candidate might be vitamin A, which acts generally fertility-promoting, probably also in parasites. The concentrations of feed supplements in the intestine as a result of feeding of fortified feeds are clearly increased compared to the concentrations which occur in the intestines of naturally fed animals.

If a deworming only with ginger should not be sufficiently successful, freshly grated **horseradish** can be given in addition (for at least 1 week in a dosage of 20 to 25 grams per 100 kilograms of body weight daily, see **part B of the book**). Also for horseradish an anthelminthic action is known. **Horseradish** has an **antibiotic effect** and kills germs what could explain this effect, because it is well known that **antibiotics** can also fight some **worm-caused illnesses** in people (e.g. elephantiasis), since worms rely on certain bacteria in their own digestive tracts and die if these bacteria are killed.

But for tapeworms even a combination of ginger and one week of horseradish has not been enough for removal of the worms. These worms seem to be especially tough! They should therefore be eliminated, as already described, with a specific drug (e.g., praziquantel).

In recent years the recommended time intervals between dewormings were constantly shortened because the worms became more and more resistant (and, as is my own opinion, horses additionally became less resistant by the "modern" kind of feeding). I would therefore advise horse owners who have problems with worms in their animals the feeding of ginger, possibly together with two deworming treatments annually. Even better is the principle of "selective deworming", which is already being used more consistently in some countries (for example, the Netherlands, Denmark) to reduce resistance in worms. About four times a year a feces sample is examined in a special laboratory for a variety of worms and then only action specifically against the worms whose egg count exceeds a certain limit is undertaken. I now practice this type of surveillance with my thoroughbred and the other horses of our little stable have joined as well. Previous studies at the Parasitological Institute of the University of Munich had shown that ginger had completely eliminated all examined 18 worm species, except tapeworms, which were then removed with a single dosage of praziquantel (Droncit®).

11.) Ginger is not effective against **infections** (at least in dried form and in the usually applied amounts)! (However, here one can use very effectively **horseradish**; see for more details in the **part B** of this book! Against **herpes infections licorice** seems to represent an interesting possibility; see for more details in **part C** of this book!) Since ginger, however, partially hides symptoms of infections, this must be taken into account (when dosages exceeding about 3 grams per 100 kilograms of body weight are fed). Thus, if difficulties occur during the feeding of ginger, bacterial or viral infections should be taken into consideration. This is especially true for dental problems, but also, e.g., for borreliosis. In some cases, it may also happen that a previously for long time unknown infection appears openly first after feeding of ginger. This is because the body tries to fight bacterial infections with the help of an inflammatory reaction, which also fights the infectious agents. By inhibiting the inflammation, the fight against the pathogens can therefore be inhibited too. This is a well-known mechanism for all anti-inflammatory agents, but it is far less pronounced for ginger than for chemical drugs!

In very large amounts of **about 25 grams per 100 kilograms of body weight, ginger** has a **strong expectorant effect**, also on toughly sticking mucus in the lung. This could be due to the content of essential oils. It seems, as if ginger also has an antibacterial effect in these large amounts. (Such an effect is described, for example, by Sebiomo et al. In the Journal of Microbioloy and Antimicrobials, Vol. 3 (1), pp. 18-22, Jan. 2011). Nevertheless, it is safer to rely on horseradish if a strong antibiotic action against harmful bacteria is needed.

I would like to emphasize that ginger (and also horseradish, see part B, or licorice, see part C) **cannot and should not replace the veterinarian!**

Ginger should only be used in higher (!) dosage for the treatment of diseases, if the **diagnosis** of the vet - or your own – is **reliable**, or the treatment concerns only **age-related diseases** in which one can only treat symptoms anyway.

However, it should be used by all responsible veterinarians for the benefit of the animals in as many cases as possible, including follow-up care to support long-term healings. Vets have substances that work faster than ginger, but I do not think they have better ones! Hence ginger is already recommended by some vets, including racetrack vets. However, the purchase of a controlled quality directly from the veterinarian is, unfortunately, still not possible.

Ginger and doping

In principle ginger, although a food, is a doping agent, if it is given in pain-relieving and anti-inflammatory amounts. That's why I had informed the Board of Thoroughbred Breeding and Racing in Germany and also the FN about it in mid-2002! For some years now it has been on the official list of drugs! However, in this list the retention time in the body is scheduled with only 2 days, which is too low! You should start leaving it away at least 4 to 5 days before a competition!

However, until it was included in the doping list, ginger (and apparently also horseradish) had long since found its way into tournament and racing sports. Especially after the case of "Renaissance Fleur" got widely known, the number of horses fed with ginger had increased dramatically and also reached other fields of horse sports. None of the usual animal studies in clinical trials could, in my opinion, be a more reliable and tougher test of value and tolerability than racetrack performance. For racing, which takes place under the most reproducible test conditions (length of the track, condition of the ground, weight to be carried, etc.), everything is meticulously recorded and repeated), it can roughly be said that ginger increases the rate of wins by about 30%.

However, in **my opinion** feeding ginger is, **depending on the amount fed**, **not** necessarily **doping**, but a **back adaptation to an evolutionary more suitable feed**! Therefore, in my opinion, a permitted limit for ingredients or metabolites of ginger in the blood should be set, because **below the threshold amount described earlier**, ginger acts no longer pain-relieving, but is only **beneficial** for the horses, it is therefore not doping but only good feed! The horses are healthier and therefore run better!

My many years of experience with ginger in horse feeding seem to show that ginger acts as a substitute with which is given back to the horse what people had taken from it once when they **domesticated** it and turned the **vagrant animal to a sedentary** one.

Something similar is known in human nutrition (European journal of Nutrition, Vol. 40, p. 289, 2002). By the use of pesticides in agriculture the content of salicylic acid has strongly decreased in plants. Salicylic acid is usually formed by plants as a protective mechanism against illness and pest infestation. In people it reduces the likelihood of heart attacks, strokes, and even cancer. People are obviously adapted evolutionary to its ingestion, and, hence, the strong reduction of the content in their today's food is associated with an increase of these illnesses. In cases of discomfort, the lack of it must then partly be compensated artificially by ingestion of acetylsalicylic acid (Aspirin®). However, nobody would have the idea to call biologically grown plants "doping"!

Also, only in recent years the **significance of spices in human nutrition** has been recognized more and more. According to the classical theory of nutrition which was based only on proteins, carbohydrates, fats, vitamins and mineral substances, they were completely negligible. However, **spices** influence **considerably**, e.g., **blood pressure**, **glucose** and **blood lipid concentrations** and **many other parameters** which are important for health! Thus, e.g., **cinnamon** reduces in people the **(bad) cholesterol values LDL** and **blood glucose** by about **10 to 30%**, already when taken in amounts ranging from 1 to 6 grams daily (Diabetes Care, Nov., 2003, Vol. 26, p. 3215) and thus has a similarly strong effect as a medication. And this without adverse side effects! (**Cinnamon** is therefore already used by some horse owners for the treatment of **Equine Metabolic Syndrome**!)

As for the beneficial effect of spices on the digestion of people, one of the acting mechanisms has been identified (Brown et.al., Gastroenterology, Vol. 132, 2007): According to this, surprisingly, receptors for some flavoring substances were found in the mucous membrane of the digestive tract, which were known before only from the nose, and which are responsible for the sense of smell. In the stomach mucosal lining, the flavoring substances provoked in these sensor cells an increase of the calcium concentration in the cytoplasma and the production of serotonin. Serotonin is commonly known as the "happiness hormone". But it also promotes intestinal peristalsis and the release of digestive juices.

The observed effects of ginger on digestion and well-being of the horse show that obviously the horse also possesses such sensory cells in the digestive tract. And the fact that horses feel so well during the feeding of ginger, might be based partially on the effect of the "happiness hormone" serotonin. Then the term "well-being dosage" could be taken quite literally.

Therefore: Food cannot be outlined with only some few parameters. It is composed of many a thousand components, many of which interact with one another.

Treatment of people and dogs

In Australia investigations are in progress concerning the use of ginger against pain and inflammations of people, which aim, however, at the chemical variation of its ingredients. But a drug based on it had to be withdrawn from the market because it was not sufficiently tolerable to the stomach. This comes as no surprise to me, because the many other additional compounds in ginger are the reason for the good tolerability of the whole plant.

In a 2010 study, ginger was also found to relieve exercise-related muscle pain in humans (C.D. Black et al., The Journal of Pain, 2010).

It is known in veterinary medicine that **most drugs work better in horses than in people**. Thus, e.g., the anti-inflammatory dosage of Aspirin® for a warmblood horse amounts to about 3 grams per day, for people which weigh much less, the dosage is 1 to 2 grams!

With ginger this relation is even more extreme. A reason for it probably lies in the fact that the **gingerols of ginger are not very resistant to acid** and people have a distinctively stronger stomach digestion than a horse, in which the stomach is less a digestive organ, than rather a "disinfection chamber" and sluice to the intestines.

For dried ginger with at least 2% of pungent substances (for ginger of African origin also a lower content of pungent substances of about 1.5% is sufficient) **dosages between 15 and 30 grams per 100 kilograms of body weight and day** were determined (by me and others too) **as necessary for mere joint illnesses of humans**. (I myself take ginger into the mouth after meals and then swallow it down with some cold milk, larger quantities I divide into smaller portions and distribute them throughout the day.)

Again, a very sudden onset of the effect was observed only after exceeding a threshold amount. This means that (when the ginger is given orally without protection against the gastric juice) **humans are about seven times less sensitive** to the analgesic and anti-inflammatory effect of ginger **than horses**!

In one case there was a report about strong flatulence as an adverse effect, however, in this case ginger (18 grams of ginger for a woman of 60 kilograms of body weight) not only helped against arthrotic pains, but even against **fibromyalgia**.

Flatulence as a side effect seems to be very rare. It is more common for high ginger dosages (more than 30 grams daily) to make feces more soft. But there is no diarrhea! With longer-term intake, the feces then becomes firm again. At very high dosages of ginger, sharpness can also be felt in urine and feces. Here, too, the body gets used to it with time. By dividing the total dosage into smaller amounts throughout the day, this side effect can also be reduced.

It has turned out that **in humans, unlike in horses** (!), the **anti-inflammatory effect** of ginger **occurs much faster**, but also **decays much faster**! For this reason alone it makes sense to divide the daily amount into several smaller amounts at different times. In **humans**, the effect generally **starts about 2 to 3 hours after intake** and begins to **subside** again **after 6 hours** . Therefore, it has turned out to be practicable to take a ginger dose in the morning, at noon and in the evening after meals. It may be possible to take another dose late at night.

Daily **8 to 12 grams** of ginger **per 100 kilograms of body weight** helped against **edemas** in the legs.

For **dogs** the necessary dosage seems to be **even a little bit higher** than for people. For **a German shepherd with 30 kilograms of weight, about 10 grams per day** must be estimated. However, **compared with horses**, **dogs** are substantially **more picky** about ginger, presumably because of the smell, which is the reason for the frequently encountered difficulty to reach the effective threshold amount. Nevertheless, on account of their strong gastric juices dogs are also able to utilize a **quite roughly cut dry ginger** which smells much less. In this state they accept it (above all in dry feed) much better. Some dog owners have also succeeded by offering ginger in cat food.

The ginger amounts required for pure joint diseases and direct administration orally (without a protective coat against the gastric juice) thus behave, **equated to the same body weight, for horse: human: dog approximately as 1: 7: 10**.

Apparently this relation can be changed for people in a favorable manner, if ginger in dry form is packed into **capsules which are resistant to gastric juice** and then have them swallowed unchewed. Thereby the decomposition process in the stomach is avoided and results in a significant increase in effectiveness.

Unfortunately capsules, which are for sale as being allegedly resistant to gastric juice, usually are not really resistant to it, but only show a somewhat delayed dissolution in the gastric juice as a result of their coating (e.g., Eudragit®). (Hence, they are called more correctly delayed-release-capsules). I have thus by myself developed capsules which extend the time until dissolution in the gastric juice to about 1 ½ hours and thereby allow a non-destructive passage through the stomach, especially, if the capsules are taken some time before the meals. That is, because in an empty stomach the passage is faster than in a full stomach. However with rich meals the stomach passage is clearly slowed down and amounts to more than 2 hours. Another method to accelerate the stomach passage is the swallowing together with carbonized mineral water: the carbon dioxide in the stomach then shortens the retention time there.

This kind of capsules is very easy to produce by oneself. They are simply **double capsules**: an outer capsule envelops and protects an inner capsule containing the ginger. Surprisingly it has turned out that such capsules, if they have a certain intermediate gap between each other, dissolve not only just twice as slowly as single-walled capsules, but much slower! Thus, e.g., commercial single-walled capsules made of hard gelatin dissolve in the stomach within about 5 to 10 minutes, single-walled vegetarian capsules (made of a substituted cellulose) dissolve even faster within about 5 minutes. However, a ginger-containing double capsule made of a hard gelatin capsule of size 0 wrapped up in a hard gelatin capsule of size 00 dissolves after about 1 to 1 ¼ hours. A ginger-containing double capsule made of a vegetarian capsule of size 0 wrapped up in a vegetarian capsule of size 00 dissolves even after 1 ½ hours, although the vegetarian single-walled capsule dissolves even faster than a hard gelatin capsule! The times of dissolution for capsules made of different materials are between these values.

The correct air gap between the two capsules seems to be decisive for the delay in the dissolution. The size 0 within an outer capsule of size 00 is a very favorable combination, also concerning the price. Depending on the type of ginger, a size 0 capsule may contain up to approximately 0.4 grams of ginger (in the case of Masterhorse granulated Nigerian ginger).

Vegetarian capsules, or those of hard gelatin, of the dimensions 0 and 00 are readily available via internet as "empty capsules". It is also worthwhile to order a manual capsule filling device (for size 0 in this case) which makes filling much easier. With such a very simple and inexpensive device, e.g. 50 filled double capsules can be produced within about 30 minutes.

Experiments with my gastric-juice-resistant double capsules have shown that the effectiveness of ginger is increased for people by about a factor 2 (to 3) as compared to the direct ingestion of ginger! Furthermore, the intake is especially suitable for people who do not like ginger, or are so ill that they would not be able to swallow it directly.

The increase in effect by the encapsulation by only about a factor of 2 (to 3), instead of the hoped-for factor 7, shows that for ginger too, as already observed for Aspirin®, horses apparently show an about 3 times higher effectiveness than people. (3 times 2,3 is about 7.)

(Of course the double capsules described here can also be used for encapsulations of other substances which are sensitive to gastric juice!)

Taking ginger in capsules is also recommended in all cases where the ginger dosages would otherwise be extremely high, e.g. in the **treatment of cancer** (see next chapter).

Another possibility to somewhat **increase** the **effectiveness** of ginger in humans seems to be, according to own experiments, the ingestion on an **empty stomach** (best in the morning some time before breakfast), suspended in a large amount of liquid which is drunk quickly. Then the ginger is passed very quickly into the intestine, without being exposed to the acidic environment for a long time.

In my my experience milk at about body temperature will allow a quick drinking without cold effects to the stomach.

By taking this on sober stomach, the effectiveness seems be to be increased by a factor of about 1.5. Thus a 65-kilogram-person with, e.g., a hip joint inflammation, does not have to eat 20 grams daily, but only 14 grams.

For an administration on an empty stomach, however, the stomach must be used to it better than would be necessary when taken right after eating!

People must in any case first **practice** the **intake** of ginger with small and slowly increasing amounts! Yet, one gets used to it quickly. The sensation of sharpness (with ginger a kind of "pseudo sharpness", because it has no harmful effects) disappears quickly (within some minutes).

A clever dog owner feeds the **ginger** to her dog with arthrosis by wrapping it **in melted cheese**! She cuts a cheese slice in two parts, melts it, then gives a teaspoon of ginger on one half, folds the other half over it and throws this cheese bag at her dog so that it devours it without chewing. The cheese apparently encapsulates the ginger reasonably well, so that the **necessary dosage drops to about one third** as compared to unpackaged ginger!

Even the dog owner herself, who also takes ginger against arthrosis, could significantly reduce the dosage of ginger she usually would need by wrapping it in molten cheese!

When ginger is administered to humans and dogs, there is still a great potential to significantly increase its effectiveness through a more appropriate and at the same time simple way of taking it!

Whether or not the effectiveness of ginger in humans (and dogs) does increase slightly by the simultaneous administration of fructose, as it does in the horse, has not been studied by me yet, but it should be worth a try!

Use of ginger against other diseases (in humans and animals)

a.) Alzheimer's disease, Parkinson's disease

A still speculative but very hopeful area of use for ginger in people could be **Alzheimer's disease**, perhaps also **Parkinson's disease**. It has already been confirmed by many large-scale research programs that **non-steroidal anti-inflammatory drugs**, even in low dosage, when offered for several years **decrease the risk** to fall ill with Alzheimer's disease **by up to 80%**! (E.g., by researchers of the Erasmus-medicine centre in Rotterdam, published in "New England Journal of Medicine", Nov., 2001, Vol. 345, p. 1515; from the University of California, published November 2001 in "Nature"; from the Universities of Toronto and Washington, American Academy of Neurology, in 2003; moreover by Herrup, Lamb et al. in "Journal of Clinical Investigation", Nov., 2009). Furthermore it was found that nonsteroidal anti-inflammatory drugs can even dissolve existing Alzheimer-plaques (J.R.Barrio et al. in "Neuroscience", issue of March 31, 2003)! New, very successful research with the anti-inflammatory acting yellow color curcumin from turmeric (also a plant of the group of ginger plants and a component of the spice curry) gives an even stronger indication that the ingredients of ginger should also be effective against Alzheimer. For curcumin a strong efficacy could be seen concerning dementia of mice, and also a reduction of existing Alzheimer plaques (Cole, J. Biol. Chem., Vol. 280, 7, p. 5892, in 2005; Fiala, Cashman, Proceedings of the Nationwide Academy of Sciences, in 2007, Vol.104, p. 12849ff). Such effects have also been suggested by studies with people (Fiala et al., Journal of Alzheimer's Disease, October, 2006). Moreover, epidemiological studies have also taken place already (Ng et.al., Am. J. of Epidemiol., in 2006, 164 (9), 898-906).
(See also the **chapter: „Turmeric as a ginger substitute?"** in this book.)
In addition, there are studies which suggest that drugs which work against Alzheimer's disease, should also be tested against Parkinson's disease (B. Gaisson et al. in "Science", Apr. 2003, Vol. 300, p. 636).
Because ginger acts just as well as a non-steroidal anti-inflammatory drug, a **positive influence** is therefore **likely on both diseases**.

b.) Acceleration of healing

A long-term feeding of ginger in already half to two thirds of the usual threshold amount for joint diseases seems to significantly **accelerate the body's healing reactions** of joints as well as of tendons and ligaments.
The externally visible ringbone at the coffin joint of my warmblood gelding, which had first built up during 7 months of acute inflammation, (he was at that time 31 years old), during which he was treated with a pain-relieving and anti-inflammatory ginger dosage and which within this time had resulted in a steeper hoof angle, had receded strongly within about 9 months after the end of the acute phase and subsequent reduction of the

ginger amount to half the dosage which does not act pain-relieving and anti-inflammatory any more. The thickening (connective tissue) at the coronet shrank during this time to about one quarter of the initial volume, and the hoof reformed itself again to its former angle and shape. The stiffening of the joint had obviously disappeared completely. An **X-ray image** which was made, unfortunately, not until 1 year after the end of the acute phase, displayed that the joint space was free again. Other X-ray images taken about 1 year and 2 years later after feeding of 2 grams or 4 grams per 100 kilograms of body weight showed no changes in the ringbone (exostosis) on the outside of the coronet bone compared with the first X-ray image. The condition of the bony outgrowth was as if frozen.

According to common experience the outgrowths would have had increased and the leg become even thicker without ginger feeding. But the contrary could be observed!

Fig.1 shows one of the **X-ray images** of the foreleg of my (in spite of strong visible exostoses) lame-free chestnut. The other ones are not different.

According to the owner of Renaissance Fleur, also with this mare a clear decrease of the perimeter around the area of the formerly smashed joint was evident after 2 years of feeding ginger at a dosage of 3 grams per 100 kilograms of body weight.

I also got reports from several other users of ginger, who confirmed this externally visible receding of ringbone at their horses during long-time feeding of ginger. One user also confirmed a radiographically verified disappearance of an ossification within the joint space during treatment of a coffin joint inflammation of her horse with ginger.

Furthermore, on the X-ray images of my gelding (32, 33 and 34 year-old at that time) an only very slight ossification of his hoof cartilage could be recognized. To what extent this is linked to the feeding of ginger, however, is not clear, because there are no X-ray images of the state, before the feeding started. I suppose that one reason for this is the fact that he received no fortified feeds and no mineral feeds. For feeding calcium together with vitamin D can result in depositions of calcium carbonate even within muscles! I am sure that an oversupply of calcium and vitamin D is one of the reasons for the nowadays so often observed ossification of hoof cartilage even in young horses.

In this context, I would also like to warn against the feeding of calcium supplements while treating the horse with Tildren® (a bisphosphonate)! Tildren® is used e.g. in case of navicular disease (podotrochlosis) to rebuild the damaged navicular bone a bit. A side effect of the treatment may be that the calcium level in the blood drops. But before calcium supplements are simply fed blindly, the calcium level should be determined during the treatment! Because I have evidence that the uncontrolled feeding of a calcium supplement leads to bony deposits not only on the navicular bone but also on other irritated sites, e.g., on tendons and in joint spaces, i.e., where you do not want such deposits!

Fig.2 shows an **X-ray image** of the left foreleg of my **English thoroughbred** Amarock (sire: Mendez, mare: Arjona out of Aggravate) at the age of 19 years. The joints are in spite of his age and 39 races (3 victories, 18 placings) still surprisingly good. Also the ossification of the hoof cartilage is only minor. Apparently, the ginger which he had received during more than 3 years before the X-ray image had had a protecting influence on the joints.

Fig.3 shows an **X-ray image** of the left hock of Amarock in April 2008 at the age of 21 years after 5 years of eating ginger. According to a vet, this X-ray image shows a joint which would even be good for a young horse!

The fact that the joints of my thoroughbred are still largely free of arthrosis even at his age could possibly be based on blocking of the protein Syndecan-4 within the joint. This protein was discovered by a research group around Prof. Pap at the university of Münster (publication in August 2009) and activates enzymes which attack the joint cartilage. By blocking Syndecan-4 the researchers could prevent the formation of arthrosis in mice.

Which ingredients of ginger and combinations of them are mainly responsible for each effect is not yet examined, however. Nevertheless, compared with the drugs usually applied by veterinarians, ginger has in my opinion the advantage of consisting of a mixture of hundreds of effective substances. Thus there is a great likelihood that there are also substances present which help the body to repair damages of a kind which the doctor had not diagnosed at all. This is a property which a good foodstuff should have. However, the big number of partially interacting substances complicates the deduction of the mechanisms of action and to establish exact criteria of quality.

Hence up to now, only the content of pungent ingredients and/or the producing country can be recommended empirically as a quality criterion.

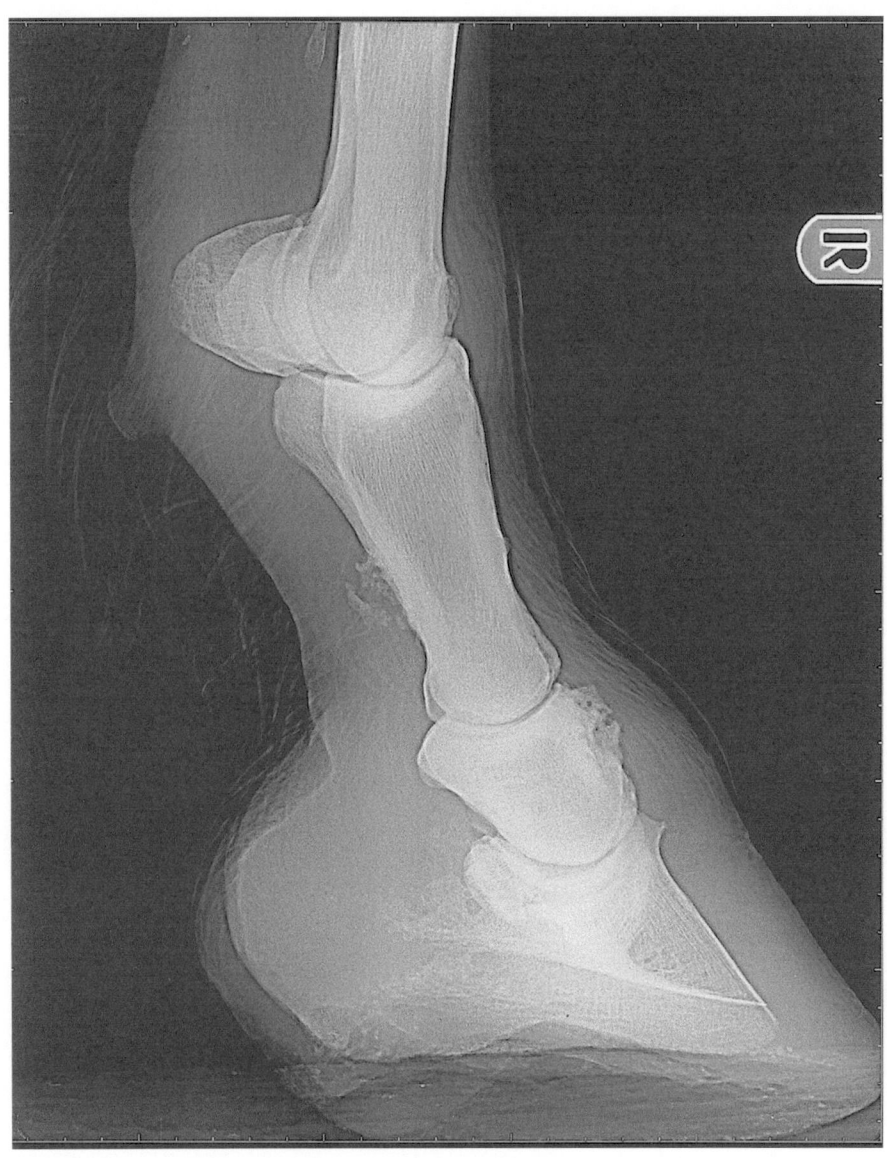

Fig.1 (Waran, right frontleg, November 2003)

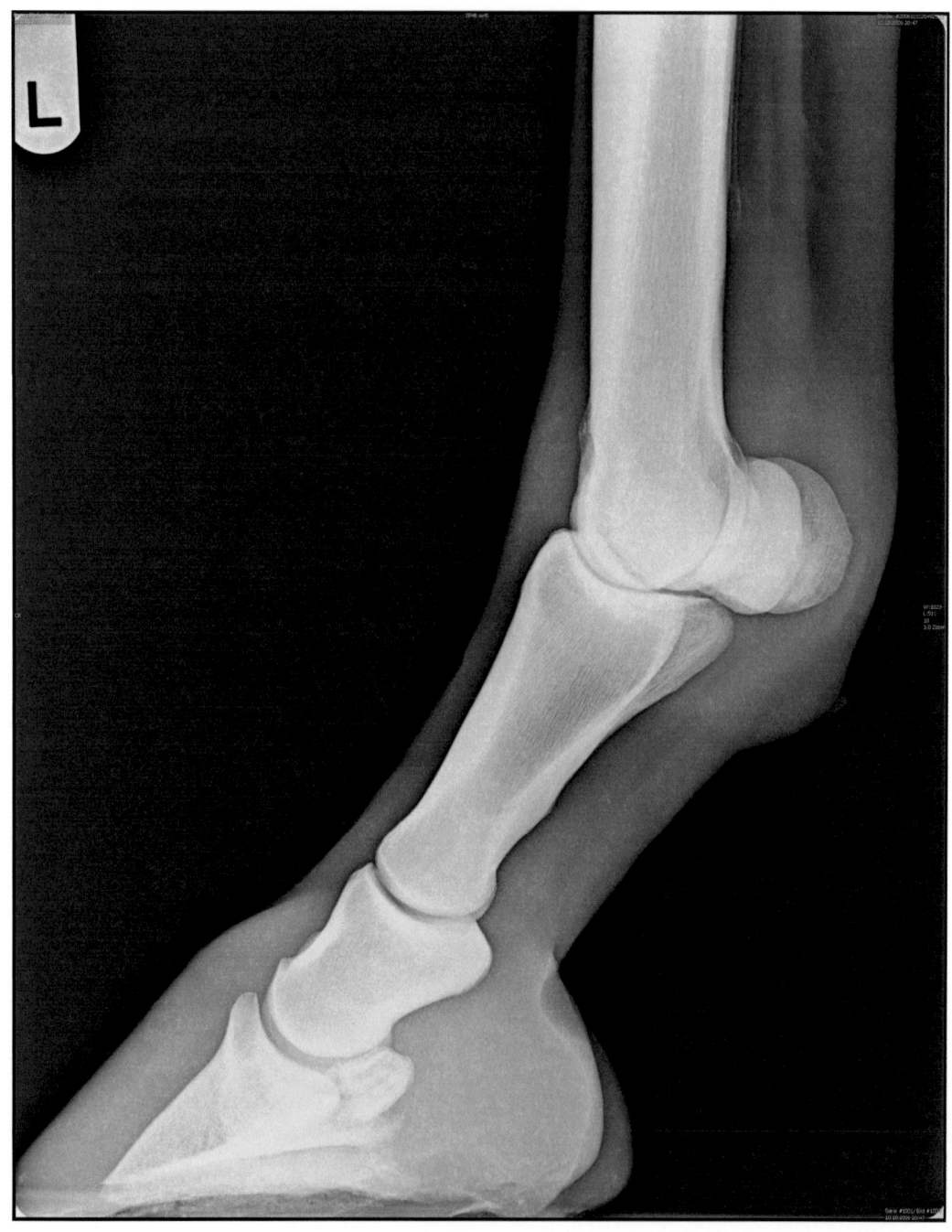

Fig.2 (Amarock, left frontleg, October 2006)

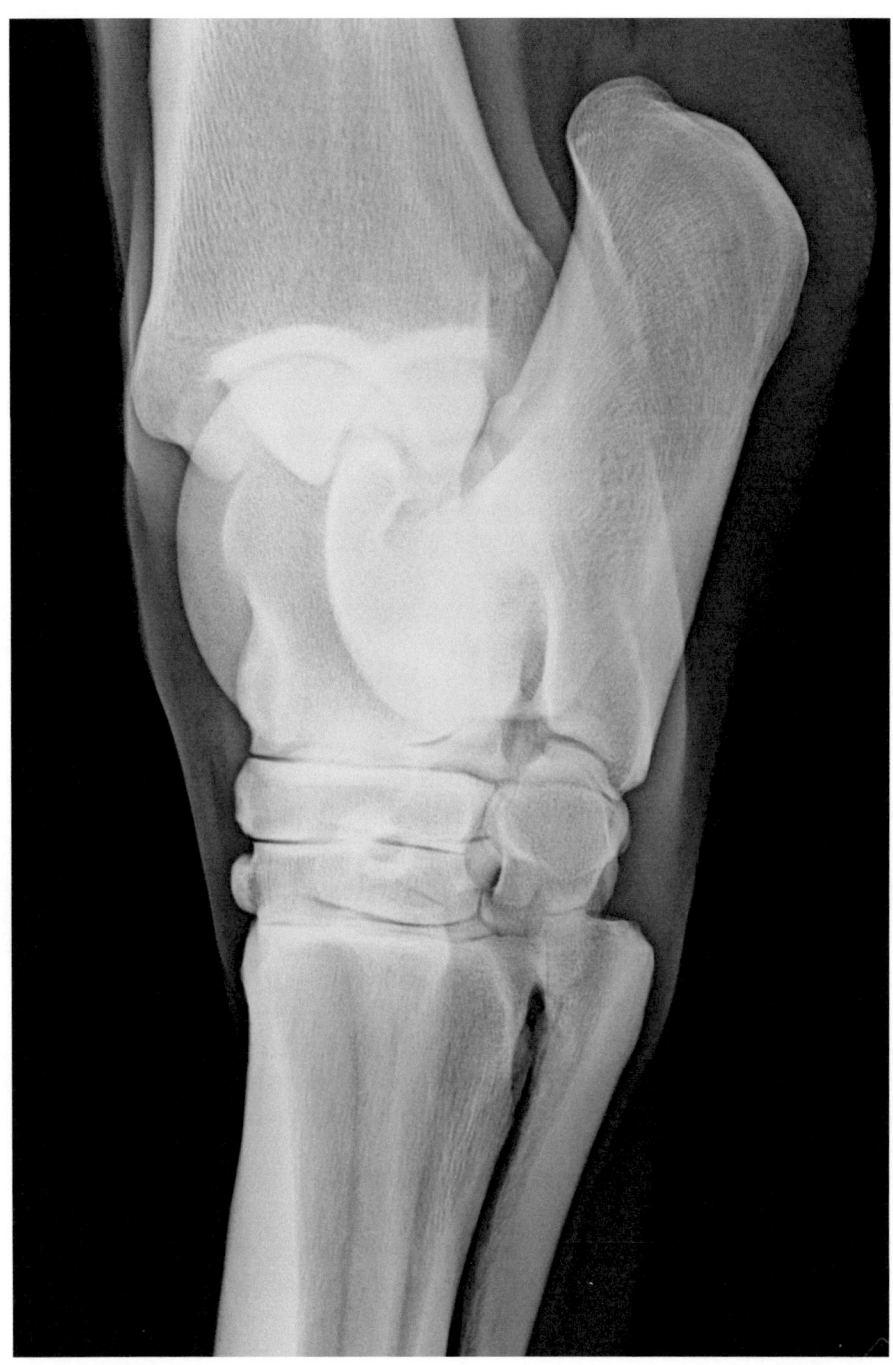

Fig.3 (Amarock, left hock, April 2008)

c.) Ginger against nausea and gastric ulcers

Ginger has long been used by people against seasickness and morning sickness during pregnancy. (Several studies have confirmed the effectiveness and safety during pregnancy: Obstetrics & Gynecology 2005 (105), p. 849-856; Midwifery, Dec. 2009, vol. 25 (6), p. 649-653).

Furthermore, a large number of **"ginger foals"** have already been born. For example even Regatta, mother of Renaissance Fleur, who receives ginger because of her melanomas (white horse), in April 2005, at the age of 25 years, gave birth to a healthy and very vital colt (Rossini). Renaissance Fleur gave birth to a filly (Roulette), fit as a fiddle, in April 2006. The next filly (Reminescence), came 2008, and another filly (Residence), in 2010. Besides, the end of feeding of the mare's "ginger milk" obviously leads to **no "withdrawal symptoms"** in the foal.

The picture from 2006 on the cover of the book shows Regatta (26 at the time of taking the picture), Renaissance Fleur (14), her filly Roulette and the proud owner of all three. Renaissance's formerly shattered and now stiff and, unfortunately, skew fetlock can clearly be recognized on the picture.

There have been reports to me about long-term feeding of up to 60 grams (total quantity) of ginger per day during **pregnancy** without adverse effects. In my opinion even positive effects are conceivable, one reason being that endoparasites are suppressed by ginger (see number 10 of the chapter "Use"). At least all foals of which I have knowledge seem to be of good health and shape.

For people aspirin and other blood-diluting medicines definitely seem to have advantages, e.g. the likelyhood of premature births and pregnancy toxicosis decreases. However, one must pay attention to the possibility of stronger bleedings (L. Askie, Lancet, May, 2007). Ginger could therefore have a comparable effect in horses, but the blood-thinning effect of ginger is low compared to that of Aspirin®.

In former times ginger was also given to make some herbs more stomach-tolerable. Also in case of **gastric ulcers**, good results were achieved in people.

A very detailed dissertation of 2006 ("Pharmakologische Untersuchungen zum Antiemetischen Wirkungsmechanismus des ätherischen Öls von Ingwer (Zingiber Officinale Roscoe)") about the antiemetic effect of ginger carried out by A. Riyazi at the Westfälische Wilhelms-Universität Münster, is freely accessible (in German) via internet at
http://www.ginger-power-company.com/diss_riyazi.pdf
or at
https://de.scribd.com/document/70221848/Dissertation-Pharmakologische-Untersuchungen-zum-antiemetischen-Wirkungsmechanismus-des-atherischen-Ols-von-Inger-Zingiber-officinale-Roscoe-von-Anj

Ginger has also proved effective for treatment of nausea during chemotherapy (even in very small amounts of about 1 gram per day (ONCOLOGY, vol.18 No.6, June 15th 2009): http://www.cancernetwork.com/nausea-and-vomiting/article/10165/1422182?verify=0

d.) Ginger for improvement of digestion and against fecal water and diarrhea

Many horse owners report about a distinct reduction of fecal water and diarrhea after feeding of ginger. An internationally much noted investigation (J. Agric. Food Chem., 2007, 55 (21), p. 8390, freely accessible via internet as a PDF under http://pubs.acs.org/doi/pdf/10.1021/jf071460f?cookieSet=1) has confirmed this observation for people, at least for diarrheas which are caused by the enterotoxin of a certain strain of Escherichia coli. Diarrheal diseases by this E. coli strain cause about 380.000 deaths of people every year! According to this research, some ingredients in ginger prevent the docking of the poisonous molecules to cell receptors, and thereby prevent diarrhea. The most important active substance for this seems to be zingerone, a substance which is generated during the aging of ginger during improper storage. Therefore in this case, old ginger might be better for treatment of diarrhea than the relatively new qualities used to inhibit inflammation! Another interesting speculation of the study: Ginger might presumably have a positive effect on cholera, because the toxin of E. coli and of cholera germs is 75% identical! (Unfortunately, this study has a great disadvantage! Coming from the „ivory tower of science", it provides only complicated information about the used essences, thus giving to country doctors in developing countries no easy, definite instructions what sort of ginger they should choose, and what the exact dosage should be!)

The veterinary practitioner Claudia Nehls has made the observation that when treating flatulence of horses with ginger, the effect is lasting for only about 8 hours, and then another dose is necessary. Hence, it could also be advantageous or necessary for the treatment of diarrhea to portion the ginger into several meals a day.

Ginger also improves digestion in general. This effect exists generally for spices in people and was examined more exactly by scientists of the University of Munich (Braun, Voland, Kunz, Prinz, Gratzl, Gastroenterology, vol. 132, 2007). With high probability the findings are also valid for horses. Accordingly, in the mucous membrane of the gastrointestinal tract, surprisingly, there are sensor cells with receptors for some of the aromatic substances which were otherwise known only from the nose and there belong to the sense of smell. In these sensor cells in the stomach mucosal lining the eaten aromatic substances lead to an increase of the calcium concentration in the cell plasma and to the production of serotonin. Serotonin is commonly known as the "happiness hormone" and leads to mental well-being. But it also enhances the motility of the intestines and the release of digestive juices.

The observed effects of ginger on digestion and well-being of horses show that obviously horses too seem to have such sensor cells in their digestive tract. And the fact that horses feel better with feeding of ginger, might be based partially on the effect of the "happiness hormone" serotonin. Therefore, the name "well-being dosage" may be taken quite literally.

The fact that ginger influences motility of bowels positively, may also be apparent from the case of a horse that came to our stable in 2006, and before that had had colics every few weeks (and also two operations). After very careful and slow heightening of the dosage of ginger it has developed no more colic since this time, although it lacks quite a piece of its bowels!

e.) Ginger as an aphrodisiac

In some countries ginger is used as an aphrodisiac for people. Such an effect seems to be given with mares at least: their **heat is enhanced**. That could make a usage in breeding reasonable for problematic mares. For this purpose, half a "joint dosage" is sufficient, that is, about 1.5 to 2 grams per 100 kilograms of body weight. I know of two mares who after many years of fruitless attempts became pregnant only after feeding ginger to them.
For stallions which are used for breeding I have no reports. However, with my geldings I could not observe any„androgenic effects".

f.) Life-extending effect

In China ginger is associated with a long life. (About the Chinese philosopher Confucius (551 –479 B.C.) is known that he ate ginger every day and in each of his meals. And even if he did not survive by this until today, at least his wisdom survived until our day!)
For horses I estimate a life-extending effect of **at least 1 to 2 years! Horseradish** helps to even **further extend** the life span in a way worth living! (See part B of this book.)

g.) Ginger against cancer

Investigations show that ginger has a marked inhibitory effect on colorectal cancer in mice that have been injected with human colon cancer cells! These mice had received half a milligram of 6-gingerol, one of the anti-inflammatory compounds of ginger, 3 times a week. (Publication by the American association for Cancer Research on October 28th, 2003)
For people, too, there are studies which attest ginger effectiveness, e.g. against ovarian cancer (J.R.Liu, University of Michigan, April 2006). Besides, it was discovered that ginger kills cancer cells not only by **apoptosis**, but also by **autophagy**. (Apoptosis is a "suicide program" of the cell, autophagy or autophagocytosis is the programmed self-degradation.)
On account of earlier references to **anti-carcinogenic effects**, I have been observing more closely the effect of ginger on **melanomas of three white horses** since the beginning of the year 2003. Melanomas are suited for this very well, especially in the early stages, because their size and number is easily recognizable externally.
For ginger dosages below the threshold amount for joint inflammation (I used 1.5 to 2 grams of African ginger with a pungent substance content of at least 2 % per 100

kilograms of body weight) the number and size of the melanomas still increased, although I cannot say whether they would have increased faster without ginger. But after increasing the dosage to **3 to 4 grams per 100 kilograms of body weight** (the "joint dosage") the **growth obviously slowed down considerably**. The **threshold amount** for joint inflammations could thus act as a threshold amount too in this case (melanomas of white horses). A horse owner even reported to me (as a side effect of the treatment of a navicular disease/podotrochlosis) a decrease of a **carcinoma** at the eyelid of her horse by about two-thirds when given 3 grams per 100 kilograms of body weight.

The dosage of 3 grams per 100 kilograms of body weight was also sufficient in my horses to significantly reduce the formation of so-called **"proud flesh"** (exuberant granuloma) in wounds!

If these results could be transferred to people, an amount of about 20 to 30 grams per 100 kilograms of body weight were to be estimated (for an oral dosage without protective sheath). (See before under „Treatment of people and dogs".)

For an 86-year-old patient with non-Hodgkin lymphoma a treatment with ginger (about 20 to 25 grams daily in fruit juice) was performed as support after a usual chemotherapy since the beginning of 2005 (G. Gennerich). By this treatment the tumor was apparently still under control after 1 ½ years, something very unusual in such a case. In a medicinal study a similar combination of usual radiotherapy or chemotherapy with simultaneous medication of commercial nonsteroidal anti-inflammatory compounds has also turned out as being more efficient than the classical single treatments (Trask, Bock, et.al., Molecular Carcinogenesis and Cancer Research, June, 2007).

I could, however, detect no influence of ginger on a malignant fast-growing **hemangiosarcoma** near the genital of my old gelding Waran, when fed at an amount of 3 to 4 grams per 100 kilograms of body weight. Thus, the effect of ginger is not the same for all kinds of malignant growths.

However, at a dosage of **around 25 grams per 100 kilograms of body weight**, ginger **removed the hemangiosarcoma** from the horse (in this case it had been Nigerian ginger with 1.6% content of sharp substances). After one week with 25 grams per 100 kilograms of body weight it had shrunk to half its size, became dry, could be ligated and dropped off permanently, which had not been possible before, when it had always returned soon afterwards. The ginger was given some more weeks, and when its amount was reduced, the sarcoma stayed away and did not return.

If the effect of ginger on human cancer were about 7 times weaker than in horses, as it is in the case of inflammations of joints, then amounts of about 175 grams per 100 kilograms of body weight would be necessary to treat an aggressive human cancer. This could hardly be achieved orally without adverse side effects, even if the amount was divided into many smaller dosages over the day! Things might look different if ginger was taken in **capsules** which are **resistant to gastric juice**, by which the effectiveness of the ginger can be increased (because of elimination of the decomposition by gastric juice). A then **still necessary dosage of 60 to 85 grams** (according to own observations the encapsulation improved the effect of the ginger only by the factor 2 to 3), **perhaps also less, per 100 kilo body weight** for several weeks or months should be well tolerated, at least it would be much (!!!) **more tolerable than chemotherapy and radiation treatment**! (For a 70-kilogram human, this would be about 42 to 60 grams, possibly less, distributed throughout the day.)

But by how much the dosage of ginger can be reduced by the use of capsules which are resistant to gastric juice cannot be predicted exactly, because it is not known whether the ingredients which are effective against cancer are the same as the anti-inflammatory ones, and whether they show a different sensitivity to gastric juice.

By the way: as to the treatment of cancer, studies with the related active compound curcumin from turmeric show also a very distinct effect on cancer of the skin (D. Siwak, Cancer, August 2005). Moreover, curcumin also prevents effectively the formation of metastases of breast cancer (Aggarwal, Clinical Cancer Research, No. 11, Vol. 20, 15/10/2005). One reason for this might be the strong inhibition of progeny of breast cancer **stem** cells, which was verified in 2009 in a tissue culture (Kakarala, Brenner et.al., Breast Cancer Research and Treatment). The concentrations required for this effect amounted to a minimum of only 10 micromoles per liter, that is a minimum of 3.7 milligrams per liter.

Anti-tumour effects are also found for intestinal cancers (Clinical Cancer Research, 12, September 2006).

Aspirin® has also been found to have an anti-carcinogenic effect (The FASEB Journal, 20, October 2006, or, specifically relating to liver cancer, J. Natl. Cancer Inst., November 28, 2012). The mechanism of acting of this nonsteroidal anti-inflammatory drug is probably based on a dosage-dependent decrease in formation of new blood vessels (inhibition of angiogenesis) within the tumor (via inhibition of a signal molecule NFkappaB), by which the tumor is starved, so to speak. Thus the non-steroidal anti-inflammatory acting ginger could also act by this mechanism, but as a multi-compound-system presumably by several mechanisms. The way in which the previously with blood much supplied hemangiosarcoma of my old gelding receded, points at least to involvement of such an inhibition of angiogenesis. For 6-gingerol, one of the pungent substances of ginger, the inhibition of angiogenesis was already verified (Biochemical and Biophysical Research Communications, Vol. 335 (2), 2005, pp 300ff).

Finally, a strong tumor-cell killing effect has also been found for the sharp substance of chili, capsaicin (T. Bates, The University of Nottingham). It is apparently based on the destruction of the mitochondria, the power stations of the cancer cells, but without affecting those of the healthy neighboring cells. In this study it was also shown that the whole group of the so-called "vanilloid" compounds, which also include the gingerols of ginger, act in the same way on the mitochondria of cancer cells: they ultimately trigger apoptosis, the suicide of the cancer cell (Bates, Biochemical and Biophysical Research Communications, 354 (1), March 2nd 2007, p. 50ff).

In a detailed article in "Spektrum der Wissenschaft" (the German version of Scientific American), issue 4/2008, has also been reported about the very **inhibiting effect of anti-inflammatory substances** on development and propagation of cancer. This article clearly states the advantages that well tolerated anti-inflammatory substances would have on development and spread of cancer. Also in a study by C. Söderberg-Nauclér et al. (J. of Clinical Investig., 2011) it is noted that many tumor cells, unlike normal cells, for unknown reasons, produce the pro-inflammatory enzyme COX-2, and anti-inflammatory substances are therefore usable for the treatment of cancer.

Since ginger is tolerated so well, it should in my opinion be a particularly suitable substance for this!

Does ginger have adverse side effects?

While ginger has been used as **food** by humans for thousands of years, it is not one of the horse-typical feeds to which the horse has adapted during the course of evolution. Hence, it was important to clarify, if there occur **adverse reactions** after long-term administration, even if these are not yet externally recognizable. Apart from the use of ginger over several years in equine competition sport, in which weaknesses would have been quickly detected, such estimates now exist for the lower dosages (of about 3 to 4 grams per 100 kilograms of body weight).

2, 3 and 4 years after the beginning of feeding ginger to my old gelding I had had blood tests taken at the age of 33, 34 and 35 years: **Neither kidney nor liver** had shown any **damage** during this time! The same is true for the blood tests of my English thoroughbred 1, 2, 3, 4, 5, 6, 7, 8, 9 and 10 years after the start of ginger-feeding. There are even reports of other horse owners that ginger had **improved** the **liver values** of their old horses.

The only "anomaly" in the blood values which I could determine for ginger-feeding was the reduction of the level of cortisol in the blood of my (at the time of those tests) 22 to 26 years old thoroughbred to levels which are typical not for old, but for very young horses. The same could be observed in a Trakehner horse of 18 and 19 years, which I had received for treatment with ginger. This could explain the easier changing of coat which even elder and very old "ginger horses" show. An explanation may be that the anti-inflammatory substances of ginger take over a part of the anti-inflammatory function of cortisol in the body, so that the body itself does not have to produce so much of it anymore. The reduction of the cortisol in the blood may also be partially responsible for the positive influence of ginger on Equine Cushing, in which cortisol levels are abnormally elevated.

Interesting in this context is that reduction of the cortisol level appears not to be linear with the dosage, but strives for a limit that seems to be about 2 µg / dl (normal value in medium aged horses: 2.9 to 9.1 µg / dl), regardless whether 4 grams or 15 grams ginger are fed per 100 kilograms of body weight. According to the investigation, this value is also reached at the latest after one month of feeding. (Furthermore, if highly-dosed horseradish is fed, the cortisol level drops even further to values of about 1.4 µg / dl.)

My own blood values of which most were within the normal limits anyhow, had, according to blood tests of 2003 and 2006, after 3 years of daily intake of ginger (3 grams for 70 kilograms of body weight) also remained constant or had become better by about 3%. There was a drastic improvement of **bilirubin**, the only one of my blood values which deviated strongly from the norm over many years (**morbus Meulengracht**, „the most unimportant disease of the world", a finding, which about 5% of the population possess without any health disadvantages). Usually the bilirubin value was within the range from 1.5 to 2.3 mg / dl, thus clearly above the norm, which considers values of up to 1.1 mg / dl as normal. After 3 years of eating ginger the value was reduced to just 0.77 mg / dl and was within the norm for the first time! At the same time the content of hemoglobin in the blood increased a little bit (bilirubin is formed in the liver by degradation of hemoglobin). However, it is possible that this drastic improvement was caused by horseradish, which I also ate in the year before the blood test (10 to 12 grams every 2 days).

Ginger dosages for different diseases of horses (table)

The table summarizes some of the observations of feeding of ginger to horses (dried ginger of African origin or Asian ginger with at least 2% content of pungent ingredients).

Remember:
Always try to eliminate or diminish the causes of a disease as much as possible!!!

	at less than 3 grams per 100 kilograms of body weight ("well-being dosage")	for more than 3 grams per 100 kilograms of body weight	for more than 6 to 10 grams per 100 kilograms of body weight
Inflammations and pain in joints in general	-	+	+
Inflammations and pain in soft tissues (tendons, ligaments, muscles)	-	-	+ (usually from 10 to 12 grams per 100 kilograms of body weight)
Navicular disease (podotrochlosis)	-	+ (for slight disease)	+ (sometimes up to 20 grams per 100 kilograms of body weight necessary!)
Diarrhea / fecal water	often +	often +	often +
Effect against worms (naturally fed horses), support by simultaneous feeding of horseradish possible	+ (within 3 to 6 weeks)	+	+
Eye inflammations	-	+	+

Cancer: melanoma (also „proud flesh")	-	+ strong growth-reduction	+
but: hemangiosarcoma (perhaps equine sarcoids)	-	-	+ (reduction of tumor beginning at about 25 grams per 100 kilograms of body weight!)
Sweet itch	-	-	? (contradictory reports)
Headshaking	-	-	- (contradictory reports)
Neuralgia (better to fight by a combination of ginger as inflammation-inhibiting agent and a pure analgesic, e.g. Traumeel®)	-	-	- (slight effect beginning at about 30 grams per 100 kilograms, possibly 80 grams per 100 kilograms body weight necessary!)
Exostoses (not too old)	(+, slowly)	+	+
Laminitis (founder)	+ (for slight disease)	+	+
Mucus liquefaction in case of sinusitis	(+)	+	+
Mucus liquefaction lung	-	-	+ (beginning at about 25 grams per 100 kilograms of body weight)
Antibiotic effect	-	-	+ (beginning at about 25 grams per 100 kilograms of body weight)

Turmeric as a ginger substitute?

As for gingerols and shogaols, a **pain-relieving and anti-inflammatory effect** is known for the active ingredient and yellow dye **curcumin** of turmeric (also a ginger plant).Therefore, there has been a lot of research on curcumin in recent years. However, turmeric has more adverse side effects compared to ginger, e.g. in larger quantities it generates nausea in people. Hence, I have only performed few tests with it.

Quite remarkable was the observation that turmeric apparently can lower the blood pressure and also relatively quickly (half an hour) after the feeding of a larger amount (about 15 grams per 100 kilograms of body weight), so that the horse stands less firmly, even lies down and then has difficulties getting up. This is not desirable in horses!

Such an effect is not observed for ginger at all, even in very high dosages. This is one reason why in my opinion one should stay with ginger and better keep one's fingers off turmeric. (For ginger, however, a moderate hypotensive effect is also observed in humans!)

But someone who owns a horse with inflammations, which gets "hot" by feeding of ginger, could also try turmeric as an alternative.

It could also be interesting for people with high blood pressure to perform the experiment on themselves. Aside from a presumably high dosage, one problem could be the rather short duration of effect, which would require very frequent intake during the day. In this case a coarser quality of turmeric could help, because it would be utilized by the body more slowly.

Frequently asked questions

Other people say, I should euthanize my old horse because I cannot use it any more, and rather buy a new one. But it is still mentally lively and happy! Shall I keep my old horse alive???

This question is practically never asked in the open, but it is certainly the one most often thought about!

Aside from the proverb „Do unto others as you would want them to do unto you!" there are, however, other reasons, why one should not simply euthanize old horses or put them down just for convenience if they still enjoy their lives.

That is because you can learn a lot by caring for an old horse and the contact with it, even for yourself! (Much more than when dealing with young horses who cope more easily with health issues resulting from mistakes.)

With horses it is not different as with people: Everyone gets older and thereby also less mobile. Nevertheless do old people still enjoy their lives and are not simply euthanized! One learns during the years to be satisfied even with less health. (Just, as one can also adapt oneself to worse external circumstances and learn to live with them.)

It is the same with horses. Horses and people do not differ very much from each other in this respect. At the same time horses are "sensor animals" that react faster and more strongly to unsuitable feed or wrong treatment than humans. (That's why there are so many sick horses in the stables.)

If you learn by observation by which simple means you are able to keep an old horse healthy and happy over a long time, you will succeed in it later also with yourself: Healthy, diverse feed which is appropriate to the species and the history of the evolution of the animal, sufficient movement conforming to the age, body weight conforming to stature and age, and social contacts.

(By the way, for people too, doctors were only in part responsible for increasing the life expectancy so markedly during the last 100 years. More than 2000 years ago in old Greece it was not substantially lower than today! Life style, hygiene (not exaggerated!) and food make up for the greatest part of it.)

For an old horse control and care of the teeth by an expert is especially important. It must also be ensured that the horse is not under stress, as can frequently be observed in herds on too small areas. Old horses should be together only with "friends", or the areas should be very large. Old horses also need to feel safe to lie down often enough, otherwise they will quickly become weak. Old horses often enjoy to lie down at noon in the safety of their box, if they can. This gives them strength again for the afternoon. A box with soft bedding offers more possibility to the old horse to lie down at night, than a place in a shared stable. For horses who have problems with getting on their legs, this is easier for them on a bedding with a grippy underground than in very cleanly mucked out boxes with concrete floor, although these are more healthy as to respiration! In very cleanly mucked out boxes with concrete floor they easily slip when getting up and then will not lie down again because of fear not to be able to get up again. (Research from 2012 also shows that properly applied mattress bedding is healthier due to the bacteria that metabolize ammonia in it than wrongly applied standard bedding!) Covering old horses keeps their muscles warm and the horses do not become stiff so quickly. Also they do not loose weight so quickly.

However, when it is not possible to remove permanent pains and illnesses from your horse any more in a simple way (e.g. with ginger and horseradish or other simple treatments), and when it is not happy any more and there is no hope for it to become happy again, and the veterinarian is a perpetual visitor to the stable, one should also in my opinion euthanize it. Then this is a true salvation. I believe no one of us would like to pine away in a nursing home and die a slow death there.

My horse does not like ginger! What can I do?

This problem crops up again and again (especially in horses that have constant access to feed in herds and do not have the necessary "ravenous hunger" to eat some strange-tasting feed for the first time). Horse owners have already tried a lot for these horses. The following possibilities were found (without claim to completeness; there are no limits to the creativity of horse owners!):

a.) Feeding in **soaked hay-/grasscubes** which **significantly reduce the sharp taste and the smell** of ginger. (This is the preferred type of feeding anyway). The hay-/grasscubes should not drip, but only have approximately the consistency of moist potting soil. This way they are better accepted by most horses! That is because the juice has a more intense and quicker contact with the mucous membranes, while the ingredients hid within the fiber are also hidden from the sense of taste.
Horses that do not like soaked hay-/grasscubes should first of all get used to aromatic, dry shredded hay-/grasscubes without ginger, and only when these are eaten with appetite, then one should begin to add more and more water and then ginger in increasing amount after the horses are used to the soaked cubes. **Addition and stirring in of ginger before the end of the soaking process** further **improves the acceptance** by the horse.
It is very useful to get horses **used to ginger**, even if they do not need it at the moment, because then in case of an emergency you will not have the problems of getting the horse used to it or of acceptance at all and can administer a therapeutic dosage immediately.

b.) Feeding ginger in a **coarser form**, in which the relative surface is lower than in a finely ground form and which therefore **smells and tastes less**. This is especially necessary for **dogs** for to reach the substantially higher body-weight-related necessary dosage for these animals.

c.) Feeding in **soaked alfalfa-cubes** which some horses like better than hay-/grasscubes. It should be noted that alfalfa is very rich in calcium and bone strengthening, but in excess can also promote ossification! The calcium/phosphorus ratio of the total daily feed must not be unhealthy! However, the feed ration of most warmbloods is more phosphorus-rich due to the grain content, so that alfalfa even partially compensates for this. Half a kilogram of alfalfa a day should therefore be completely uncritical for the vast majority of warmblood horses!

d.) **Dividing** the amount of ginger **into several portions** throughout the day in concentrated feed.

e.) Simultaneous administration of **fruit shreds**, particularly of **citrus fruits**. **Mashed bananas, grated apples or carrots** also seem to mask the taste and smell very well. **Linseed slime** (for example, in soaked hay-/grasscubes) also makes ginger palatable to picky gourmet horses.

f.) Addition of **brewer's yeast**; especially if the horse already knows the smell of it.

g.) Addition of **apple juice** or **orange juice**

h.) At first **getting the horse used only to freshly grated horseradish**, which most horses love. And then **under the "guise" of horseradish, slowly start ginger feeding** and then slowly reduce the horseradish after reaching the required ginger dosage.

i.) First, f**eed fresh, juicy ginger** (as a root) to get the horse used to the taste. Fresh ginger is usually better accepted. However, it is more expensive (you also pay for the water in it!) and usually much worse and more varying in quality.

j.) A creative owner of a "gourmet pony" has successfully tested the following: She mixed 50 grams of ginger powder with 500 grams of oak flakes and little water to get a thick mash, added sweetener (because of the teeth) and then dried this mass after spreading on a baking tray on the tiled stove (at estimated 50°C). Her pony liked these dry **oat/ginger biscuits** very much!
At this temperature the effectiveness of ginger should still not decrease much. However, instead of sweetener one could give raisins a try, because these (at least with people) – just like the sweetener - have no damaging effect on the teeth, but even, despite their sweetness, have an anti-bacterial effect on caries bacteria! Moreover, the ginger concentration in the biscuits could be increased by use of a coarser ginger form. As a sweetener one could also try licorice or fructose.

k.) Very simple and very often successful is also the mixing of **fruit sugar** (fructose) into the soaked hay-/grasscubes. Fructose ("diabetic sugar"), unlike conventional sugar or glucose, does not increase blood sugar levels and thus **does not produce sudden**

peaks of insulin levels. The hormone insulin is an endogenous compound that promotes inflammation when in excess! For every gram of ginger 1 to 2 grams of fructose are recommended. Up to 100 grams of fructose daily are considered to be completely uncritical for a large horse. This amount is e.g. already contained in a bit more than one kilogram of sweet apples!

l.) If everything else fails: Mix the ginger in good edible oil (such as thistle oil) or water/fruit juice and administer the mixture/suspension with a big syringe/dispenser directly into the mouth (similar to deworming). (Oil is presumably better, because fat generally binds sharpness.) After a while many horses will get used to getting the spicy mixture. However, at the same time one should also try to mix the ginger in very low amounts into the concentrated feed (e.g., using methods, as described above) and then increase this amount **very** slowly. If the horse realizes that ginger is good for him, it will, after some time, usually accept it also in its feed.

Is it possible to feed ginger to pregnant mares or to those that shall be mated, and what influence does the milk of such a "ginger mare" have on her foal?

There are not many empirical data known to me concerning horses. However, studies with people show that ginger has **no adverse side effects** (Obstetrics & Gynecology in 2005 (105), p. 849-856).

Already in 2005 Renaissance Fleurs mother Regatta had given birth to a very vital "ginger foal" (Rossini) which drank ginger milk and prospered splendidly. At that time she received about 3 grams of ginger powder per 100 kilograms of body weight, because of her melanoma. A year later, Renaissance Fleur also got a filly (named Roulette, sired by the stallion Summertime) without problems, which also developed splendidly with ginger milk. Because of her accidental arthrosis in the stiff right fetlock joint, Renaissance Fleur also receives 3 grams of ginger powder per 100 kilograms of body weight. (Regatta, Renaissance Fleur and Roulette are shown, together with her owner on the book cover.) In 2008, Renaissance got another beautiful filly (this time sired by Kaiser Wilhelm), which received the name Reminiscence. And in 2010, Renaissance got a filly once more (named Residence, this time sired by Hibiscus).

A horse owner I have knowledge of, gave even 10 grams per 100 kilograms of body weight to his mare without problems after the mating. A high-class mare in S-contest jumping in a neighboring stable received before, during, and after pregnancy 4 to 5 grams of ginger per 100 kilograms of body weight as well as 30 grams of horseradish per 100 kilograms of body weight, and the filly also developed splendidly.

My expectation is that "ginger foals" should develop even better and be "tougher" than those which are intensively fed with supplements, because ginger influences the digestion positively and holds down parasites. But only the coming years, when these horses get into the sport, will show if this proves to be true. At least Renaissance Fleur's offspring have all been awarded prizes.

My horse has joint arthrosis and I already feed 4 grams of ginger per 100 kilograms of body weight and still can not see success, in spite of giving the horse a break. What can I do?

If the ginger is of good quality (African or/and at least 2% content of sharp substances), it is very likely that the diagnosis has not been complete or even wrong and the reason of the lameness is another or an additional one. If there is a joint affected, not seldom the surrounding "soft tissue" (tendons, ligaments) is affected too, requiring substantially higher ginger dosages. In this case the dosage should be increased further until a clear effect occurs (often at about 10 to 15 grams per 100 kilograms of body weight). This dosage should then be given for several weeks (in the hope that the superimposed soft tissue inflammation will abate strongly during this time), before making a first attempt to lower the dosage again. A lowering of the dosage should take place most favorably during cool weather.

If ginger amounts of more than 15 grams per 100 kilograms of body weight do not show distinct improvement in spite of giving the horse a break, it is likely that neuralgia is involved (e.g. a pinched nerve in the back) or an exostosis is constantly inducing inflammation again. In this case it makes sense to administer a pure painkiller (analgesic) for some time in addition to ginger, which is primarily an anti-inflammatory agent. In my opinion in this case a good choice without adverse effects is Traumeel® , which is administered in the feed or, in little honey, with the mouth syringe directly into the mouth (about 100 drops, according to about 5 milliliters, per 100 kilograms of body weight). Another possibility, in addition to the anti-inflammatory ginger, is Novalgin® (Novacen®, metamizol) in a dosage of about 10 to 12 milliliters per 100 kilograms of body weight in the feed.

Because it cannot be taken for granted that a **pinched nerve** gets free by itself again, I strongly advise in this case to have an **osteopath** treat the horse additionally!

An **abscess in the hoof** is another reason, why high dosages of ginger show only little effect. Incidentally, hoof abscesses also react badly to conventional veterinary painkillers. In this case it is necessary to find and open the abscess.

Sugar-containing feeds and those with very easily digestible carbohydrates (e.g. bread!) also reduce the effectiveness of ginger, because they apparently promote inflammations (possibly due to increased insulin secretion)! This is probably the case in horses with Equine Metabolic Syndrome. On the other hand, fructose, which I had previously proposed as a means of making ginger tastier to picky "gourmet horses", sometimes even seems to slightly increase the effectiveness.

Is feeding of ginger doping?

See chapter: Ginger and doping, page 30.

I would like to deworm my horse with ginger. What do I have to keep in mind?

The present experiences show that in case of an only slight affliction with worms an amount of 1.5 to 2 grams of ginger per 100 kilograms of body weight for 3 weeks is sufficient. In case of a strong affliction with worms, about 6 weeks are necessary. The investigations took place in 15 naturally fed horses (no fortified feed!), and according to excrement tests all animals were free of worms after the treatment. (For sheep and dogs there exist already clinical studies on the gentle and successful deworming with ginger. (Iqbal et.al., J. Ethnopharmacol., 2006, 106, p. 285 ff.))

Later studies in the years 2010 to 2012 now give a slightly more differentiated picture : Excrement tests at the Institute for Parasitology and Tropical Medicine in Munich were examined for 18 different worm species, and the ginger seems to banish all these worms with one exception: tapeworms! Against tapeworms, therefore, should be given a specifically acting agent, when detected. One such substance is praziquantel which is the single agent, for example, in Droncit®.

Whether or not very high dosages of ginger can also drive out tapeworms has not yet been investigated. Previous research only covered long-term dosages of up to 5 grams per 100 kilograms of body weight.

The described observations refer to an African ginger with a high content in pungent substances (at least 2%) and essential oils (about 2%). However, this does not mean that other ginger kinds would not be better (but also could be worse), if, for example, quite different ingredients should be responsible for the deworming effect. There are, unfortunately, still no empirical values available.

In any case, one should have a fecal sample for safety reasons after the ginger treatment, because I have been reported cases in which the ginger has not been sufficient. There are such cases, however, also with conventional dewormings. Ginger is a mild-acting remedy which can already be recognized by the fact that it needs a relatively long time for its effect. (It is a food and no poison!) If worms find especially favorable living conditions in certain horses (e.g. because of certain supplements in fortified feed: vitamin A could play a major role here), or if the constant intake of new worm eggs is very high, then the anthelmintic effect of ginger may sometimes be insufficient to prevail against such "worm-favorable" conditions. However, in such cases an additional feeding of antibiotically active horseradish (20 to 25 grams per 100 kilograms of body weight) for about one week might enforce the anthelmintic effect.

For the worm-caused sickness elephantiasis of people (The Lancet, 365, May, 2005) and worm-caused sicknesses in the eyes it is known, e.g. that these can be treated well with antibiotics, because these kill bacteria, which are necessary for their survival, in the bowels of the worms. Besides, such a therapy fights, in contrast to many usual dewormers, not only the larvae, but also the adult worms themselves.

My horse is young and has actually no health problems. May or should I still feed ginger as a "preventive"?

If the horse is young and healthy, I personlly would not do so, because one should not make life unnecessarily complex to oneself. „A horse needs hay, oat, straw and salt!" a professor of my former veterinarian mentioned a little bit provocatively to his students. Well, grass should be there too.

Since the performance of horses increases with ginger (as one could observe on the racetracks), it is also to be feared that less experienced horse owners work the horses stronger then would permanently be good for them, and then the positive effects would be destroyed again or even overcompensated.

But if the horse is older or if a young horse already shows health problems (which are reasonably reliable diagnosed), you should not hesitate long but in my opinion start the feeding of ginger. At the beginning many wear and tear illnesses can be treated much better and faster and even heal out, as when the damage is already large.

In any case, I think it makes sense to get **all** (!) horses, whether young or old, used to the taste of ginger quite early and without stress!

By doing so you do not have to struggle with eventual acceptance problems later on, but can increase the dosage of ginger very quickly to the necessary amount! (The same goes for horseradish!)

Also a gentle getting-used to soaked hay-/grass cubes as a good and healthy "hiding place" for ginger makes sense. As soon as the horse accepts the soaked cubes with pleasure, one can stop feeding them, until one needs them again for the purpose of feeding ginger.

Does ginger work for all horses?

As to my own observations, ginger has up to now worked in all cases, IF (!) inflammations of joints or soft parts were the causes of the discomfort and the owners fed ginger in the amount necessary for the treatment of the respective disease (!) and did not stop too early, because they regarded it as too sharp for their horses. Sometimes it only turns out while feeding ginger, whether the horse has a pure arthritis or, in addition, a soft tissue inflammation. In the first case the dosage at which a sudden marked improvement begins to show, is about 3 grams of a good quality per 100 kilograms of body weight (the individual range may stretch from 2 to 4 grams). A sudden improvement usually starts with a 1 ½ to 2-day delay after the threshold amount has been reached or exceeded, so it does not take weeks! (In principle it is like the action of a classical drug, just better adapted to the body than usual drugs, which have only one active ingredient! Much as a hand can grip better than a single big finger.)

In the second case of pure soft tissue inflammations (tendons, ligaments, muscles) the threshold amount is about 10 to 12 grams (sometimes 15 grams) per 100 kilograms of body weight and day. However, I know of a 700-kilogram horse, which required a daily total of 120 grams of ginger a day for the treatment of his podotrochlosis, so almost 20 grams per 100 kilograms of body weight.

If 4 grams per 100 kilograms of body weight are not sufficient for treatment, one can be very sure that it is not a pure arthritis of joints one has to deal with!
In the "gray area" of 4 to about 8 grams per 100 kilograms of body weight it can be assumed that it is only a slight irritation of soft tissue, e.g. a tendon which rubs at an exostosis, but which is not or not yet severely inflamed.
However, for strong pure **nerve irritations** (e.g. a pinched nerve), **nerve damages** and also for **torn muscle fibers**, **ginger has not sufficient power** to significantly relieve the resulting pain. **Ginger is almost exclusively an anti-inflammatory** and is only a little bit a direct painkiller! The necessary dosage for such cases would be 60 or more grams per 100 kilograms of body weight and thus exceeds the acceptance of most horses by far! (However, in such cases in humans often even opiates do not help!). (In the case of pinched nerves, therefore, an osteopath should always be used additionally!)
In addition to the administration of ginger, the horse should **not do much work**, because existing inflammations flare up again and again, of course! (If you hit your finger with the hammer over and over, you can take whatever you want, it will never heal!)
And **no feed** should be given **which promotes inflammation**. This includes e.g. bread. If it should be all feeds with very easily digestible carbohydrates (high glycemic index), then you have to take care with such feeds too, for example molasses or grass which is rich in fructan.
In addition, in cases where high amounts of ginger are needed, a horseradish cure of at least one week is recommended to rule out an infection as a possible cause of the inflammation (see part B of this book).

Quick guide for feeding of ginger to horses

Ginger against inflammation and for pain relieving

1.) Start feeding slowly, beginning with a total quantity of about 1 gram (dry quality, preferably of **African** origin (e.g. Nigerian from the company Masterhorse), or with at least 2% content of pungent substances) per day. Preferably feed in soaked (not dripping but "earth-moist") hay-/grasscubes (choose qualities which are rich in fiber structure!), which strongly reduce the taste and smell of ginger. Then daily increase to 3 grams, then 6 grams, then 9 grams, ..., eventually faster, if the horse shows no acceptance problems, but more slowly, if kidney problems exist, or if the horse generally shows problems (such as colic) when changing feeds.
If the horse is already accustomed to ginger, you can rise the dosage very fast to the supposed necessary dosage, usually even immediately.

2.) Increase the daily total amount, e.g. in 3-gram increments, until a sudden improvement is evident. For pure joint inflammations this amount is usually about 3 to 4 grams per 100 kilograms of body weight, that is, a horse weighing 500 kilograms needs about 15 to 20 grams. (Nowadays, however, most horses weigh clearly more than 500 kilograms!)
For soft tissue inflammations (tendons, ligaments) the dosage needed to reduce inflammation and pain is usually about 10 to 15 grams per 100 kilograms of body weight, thus 50 to 75 grams for a horse weighing 500 kilograms. (For higher necessary ginger dosages one has to increase the quantity faster than in 3-gram steps, e.g. in 5-gram or even bigger steps.) The values given are guidelines and vary somewhat from horse to horse.
In about 500 grams of dry hay-/grasscubes about 20 to 30 grams of ginger powder can be given quite agreeable to most horses, in case of good acceptance or use of a coarser ginger form (such as fine cut or granular) also significantly more.
For a quantity of 100 or more grams of ginger per day, a distribution into several portions is preferred, but not absolutely necessary, especially if the ginger is served in a coarser form and in a sufficiently large amount of feed (preferably hay-/grasscubes).

3.) Then maintain the necessary dosage found for anti-inflammatory action and pain inhibition for about 4 weeks. (For very strong inflammations of the hoof joint a dosage of about to 3 to 4 grams of ginger per 100 kilograms of body weight must sometimes be given still longer, e.g. for half or three quarters of a year!)
During this time exercise the animal only in the way the vet suggests or would suggest!
If a dosage of significantly more than 3 to 4 grams per 100 kilograms of body weight had to be given, you may attempt to lower the dosage to about 3 to 4 grams per 100 kilograms of body weight after this time. If this is not possible without aggravation, the higher dosage must be maintained.

You should not try to lower the amount too soon, and also not to work the horse too soon again. If there are no kidney problems and ginger is accepted well enough by the horse, the tolerability of ginger without side effects can be trusted up to high amounts of 30 grams per 100 kilograms of body weight over a period of at least 6 to 8 months when administered in a coarser form, e.g. fine cut, in a sufficiently large amount of soaked hay-/grasscubes and when the amount is increased slowly.

However, if acceptance problems should appear, one should search for the underlying cause (e.g. sores in the mouth, gums, …).

4.) Reduction of the ginger amount to a "well-being dosage" of 1.5 to 2 grams per 100 kilograms of body weight, as soon as the affected part is no more warmer, than the corresponding one on the healthy limb.

This amount should be fed preferably for at least one to 2 further months, in the case of serious injuries, or an age of more than 15 years, better permanently.

Horse owners, who are well versed with the tolerable work load of horses, can also feed 3 to 4 grams of ginger per 100 kilograms of body weight as a lasting "well-being dosage".

5.) The table in the chapter „Ginger dosages for different diseases of horses" summarizes some of the observations about the feeding of ginger.

B. Horseradish in horse feeding

Horseradish, freshly (!) grated, in an amount (appoximate value!) of about 20 to 25 grams per 100 kilograms of body weight is an effective **broadband antibiotic** in horses against grampositive and gramnegative bacteria, e.g. in case of phlegmon (by streptococci), but also suppuration of the jaw and the like. (For severe infections you choose higher dosages for safety!)

The **effect** is already noticeable about **one day** after the feeding has reached the therapeutically necessary dosage! Of course wound care must be performed nevertheless! In case of wounds which have constant contact with dirt (especially in the lower leg area!), these must also be protected from further access of dirt (e.g. by easily applied glued-on dressings, which are also described in this book). In the hoof area where this is not possible, a shoe-formed soaked or dry absorbent cotton bandage is applied.

(You can find pictures of the horseradish treatment of a light to medium phlegmon of my thoroughbred in part A of the book about feeding of ginger (see the sub-chapter "Use", section 6); beneath this phlegmon there was additionally a soft tissue inflammation which was recognized only later and which heals better by ginger treatment; this is why the exemplary photos were depicted in part A of the book. The wound in the upper area of the cannon bone is effectively protected from dirt and flies by a glued-on dressing.)

For a **very serious phlegmon** during which the skin was already tearing and the horse could not be helped even in a clinic, according to the observation of the owner feeding of **35 grams of horseradish per 100 kilograms of body** weight with **simultaneous administration** of **5 grams of ginger per 100 kilograms of body weight** (for reduction of inflammation) were needed!

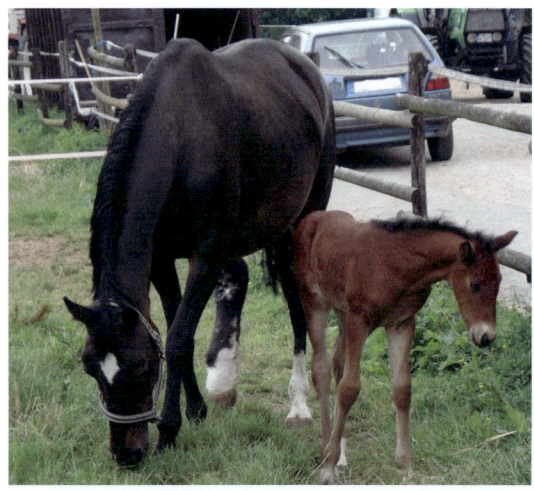

The adjacent picture shows a high-quality mare (placed in S-jumping, but otherwise quite "clumsy"; she injured herself constantly!) which during several years of unsuccessful conventional treatment had developed strong phlegmons and therefrom excessive growth of connective tissue to form an "elephant's leg" at which the skin ripped over and over again (the scars are recognizable on the picture). A use in breeding had failed because the mare did not become pregnant. After treatment with ginger (about 5 grams per 100 kilograms of body weight daily) and horseradish (about 35 grams per 100 kilograms of body weight daily) the circumference of the leg reduced to the size of the old connective tissue, the mare got pregnant and foaled a healthy filly at the age of 17 years.

Already in lower dosages of about **10 to 12 grams per 100 kilograms of body weight** horseradish eliminates those **dental infections** in the mouth, which are directly accessible for its active ingredients. Moreover, in this amount it often helps against **coughing**. (Horseradish was therefore already used by some North American Indian tribes, such as the Cherokees, against **tooth decay** and **bronchitis**!)

A **horseradish cure** every few weeks for about one week benefits **old horses** very much. After having "cleaned out" the horse with a daily amount of 20 to 25 grams per 100 kilograms of body weight, for the repetitive cures daily amounts of only 10 to 12 grams per 100 kilograms of body weight are usually sufficient.
After having performed an initial cure with 20 to 25 grams per 100 kilograms of body weight per day, you can alternatively also give the horseradish e**very week**, and then **on two or three consecutive days** (daily 10 to 12 grams per 100 kilograms of body weight are usually sufficient). I myself usually use it for horses three days a week, once in the middle of the week, the other two times on the weekend days. In my opinion, this method is also recommended for younger horses as a preventive measure. For horses that often have problems with tooth infections, the "dental dosage" should be given daily.
However, the regular use over years seems to diminish the efficacy somewhat, so that in case of a suddenly appearing infectious disease (e.g. phlegmons) higher dosages must then be given.
According to my own observations the necessary dosages increase by about 30% compared to the aforementioned amounts and thus not dramatically. (However, these dosages are still very well tolerated, which is why you should not abstain from a permanent feeding to old horses.) Presumably the reduced effectiveness is due to an increased excretion or quicker degradation by the body and not to an increased resistance of the germs. Conventional antibiotics, fed over such a long time, would have completely lost their effectiveness at the end!

The feeding of horseradish increases the **life expectancy** of old horses significantly! The fight against the dental infections which occur with increasing age and which (also for people) lead to secondary damages in the body, probably has a major influence. (See also the short report about the 109-year-old Count von Waldeck at the end of the chapter!)
Since I myself take horseradish every other day in an amount of about 10 grams (in small pieces with very little milk slowly chewed in the mouth), I have e.g. no more problems with a before rather large **periodontal pocket** at a slanted wisdom tooth! During the past 7 years, in which I practice this, my periodontal pockets have now almost completely disappeared!)
A striking feature in the feeding of horseradish to old horses (in combination with ginger, but presumably also without) is the significant and rapid **weight gain** without getting more feed! The effect may be comparable to the feeding of antibacterial substances during pork rearing. There, increase in weight is accelerated by feeding of such compounds (formerly unfortunately antibiotics, today, also unfortunately, antibacterial

copper compounds). Presumably this happens by **eliminating smaller infections** that slow down the growth of the animals.

Hence, also in the meat production for people one could in my opinion pass over to the effective and at the same time healthy horseradish!

By the way, the word horseradish has this etymology also in German. In the German word "Meerrettich" the first part of the word presumably comes from marha, Germanic for horse, which has survived in the German language as "Mähre", the English word "mare" and the Icelandic word "meri" for the female horse.

Though there are still other etymological derivations for the word horseradish, those who have experienced how much most horses almost love the grated horseradish, surely have no more doubt about the given derivation of the word.

Since horses like to eat horseradish already after a short time of getting used to it (some even pure!), the continuous raising of the dosage is mostly no problem. On the first day you often can already give 20 grams to a normal sized warmblood, the next day 50 grams, then 100 grams and then the therapeutically necessary dosage (if this should not be reached with a total quantity of 100 grams yet).

To horses which already know horseradish, you can feed the therapeutically necessary dosage immediately in case of an emergency. Therefore, as with ginger, getting the horse used to horseradish is advisable, even if at the moment there should not be acute need for it.

The horseradish must be **freshly grated** or **stabilized by an acid** (e.g. citric acid or cider vinegar), because some of its **active ingredients**, which are formed from precursor substances only after destruction of the cell walls (e.g. **allyl mustard oil** from sinigrin) are not very stable and already decompose relatively quickly in the presence of water. Some horse owners also use with success **commercial over-the-counter grated horseradish out of the glass** (not the cream containing variant!). However, it contains preservatives and the **necessary dosage is distinctly higher**. An experiment with a coughing horse proved need for about **1.5 to 2 times the amount of what would have been necessary of freshly grated horseradish**. It makes sense, always to have a big glass of commercial grated horseradish in the stable, just for emergencies if there is at the moment no fresh horseradish at hand! Moreover, I always have frozen chunks of horseradish in the freezer compartment, because horses like the frozen better than the one from the glass! The horseradish must be grated in the frozen (!) state and fed immediately. The effectiveness of frozen horseradish also is lower than that of fresh horseradish: it should be dosed about 30 to 50% higher than the fresh one. The reason may be that with freezing the developing ice-crystals already damage the cell walls (hence, it is rubber-like after thawing!) and the active substances then by and by decompose during thawing and make the thawed horseradish somewhat less effective. Horseradish is also available as a dry powder, but this seems to be even less effective in terms of dry matter than horseradish from the glass. But the degree of effectiveness is certainly very much dependent on the manufacturing procedure! A grade which I used for testing seemed, compared relative to dry matter, to be at least about 4 times less effective against cough, than the freshly grated horseradish! This could be different with other infections, however. As mentioned, the differences in quality can be huge here, however. For example, in the (German) over-the-counter human medicine Angocin®, horseradish is also included as a powder and nevertheless has a good effectiveness.

Because my (in 2013) 26-year-old English thoroughbred receives freshly grated horseradish three times a week anyhow for keeping his teeth and gums healthy, I make sure that I always have at least three pieces of suitable size for this purpose in the stable. This can be done because horseradish stays sufficiently fresh over such a time span even without cooling. In emergencies, e.g. injuries, I can then immediately grate all three pieces at once and give them as an antibiosis or I can also borrow the horseradish to other horses who need it!

The horseradish is preferably given **in one serving a day**, because some of its active compounds (**mustard oils**) are **volatile** (high vapor pressure) and are **quickly excreted by the body**, also exhaled through the lungs. If, on the other hand, the horseradish is distributed in small portions throughout the day, it is however not sure that the minimal effective concentration in the body is reached at all, because the body has long since begun to excrete the previous small dosage before the next one is fed.
Just like ginger, you feed the freshly grated horseradish very advantageously **in soaked hay-/grasscubes**.

Horseradish complements ginger in an almost ideal way! While ginger attenuates the inflammation, horseradish at the same time eliminates germs as a possible cause of the inflammation.
It may also be fed **for many weeks**. (It is also recommended to do so for complete healing of some kinds of diseases, e.g. suppurations in the jaw!). By feeding of 25 grams per 100 kilograms of body weight during up to 8 weeks (in soaked hay-/grasscubes) I myself have not encountered any problems. By contrast, when administering a conventional antibiotic for 8 weeks, serious side effects would be expected!
For a big carthorse stallion I was able to observe the feeding of 50 grams of horseradish per 100 kilograms of body weight for more than 2 months. This amount had been divided into two portions a day. A blood analysis was not made, but externally the horseradish did show no negative effects, the stallion became even stronger with time. Even amounts of more than 50 grams per 100 kilograms of body weight have been fed (in soaked hay-/grasscubes) to a pony with borreliosis for several months.
The fact that the stallion became stronger over time, does not not astonish me anymore, since in 2012 there was growing evidence that a **longer-term** (one month) **feeding** of horseradish in a dosage of about 30 grams per 100 kilograms of body weight **increased** the amount of red blood pigment (**hemoglobin**) in the blood significantly. The increase (10 to 20%!) was doping relevant, similar to EPO! I have yet to find a simple explanation for it, especially since a short-term feeding or a small dosage has no effect on the

hemoglobin level or even slightly reduces it! Does it in high dosage remove germs that are blood-destroying? Or is the reason an overreaction of the body to an initial degradation? (One could then ask oneself, if the feeding of garlic, of which was warned by media because of alleged degradation of the blood pigment, in the long term could not also lead to a similar increase in the hemoglobin level!)

However, for **humans** it is known that a **lasting (!) intake in large quantities** (more than 20 grams per day, that is **more than about 30 grams per 100 kilograms of body weight**) may lead to the formation of **peptic ulcers**. Otherwise, people do not eat horseradish in a better tolerable form in soaked hay-/grasscubes.

Still, it is more safe not to use horseradish in high dosages for years as a permanent feed, like ginger, but only at intervals.

Ginger as a **stomach-friendly** agent probably improves the **tolerability** of horseradish in long-term, high-dosage treatments. Linseed slime is also recommended for such long-term treatments.

In a recent study, an infestation of the corium of horses with laminitis with certain (mainly gram-negative) bacteria was found. („Chronic laminitis is associated with potential bacterial pathogens in the laminae", Onishi u.a., Vet. Microbiolog., 17. Aug 2012) . This finding makes it advisable to test horseradish also on horses with laminitis.

In October 2012, my then 25-year-old thoroughbred suffered from a suppuration of a tooth in the upper jaw, including fever. (He's been a crib-biter since I got him (19 years ago) and therefore does not have good teeth!) The teeth were rasped by the vet, but I treated the infection with horseradish (35 grams per 100 kilograms of body weight daily, for a month, on the first two days he even received 55 grams per 100 kilograms of body weight, divided into two portions).

The effect began almost exactly after one day, and after three days the cheek had been normal again for outsiders and the fever had gone.

Since the cause, the diseased tooth, was not removed, I continued to feed a low dosage of 12 grams per 100 kilos of body weight for a further 3 months after completion of the high-dosage treatment to allow for at least partial healing of the root of the tooth.

The pictures on the left show the condition on the first day of suppuration (11.10.) And on the right after 5 days of treatment with horseradish (16.10.):

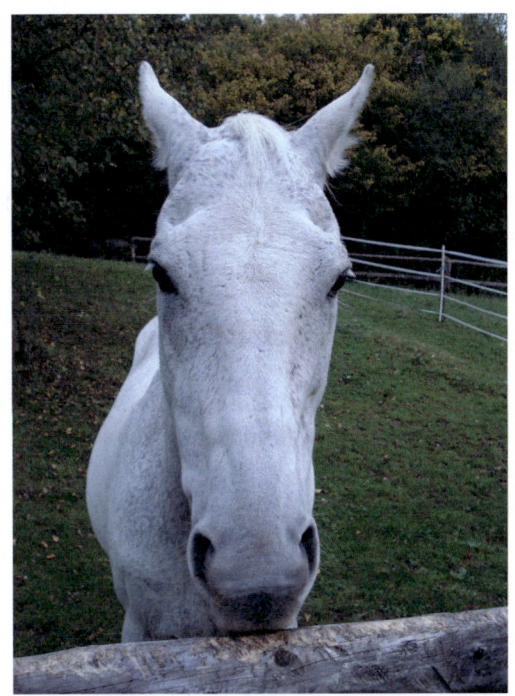 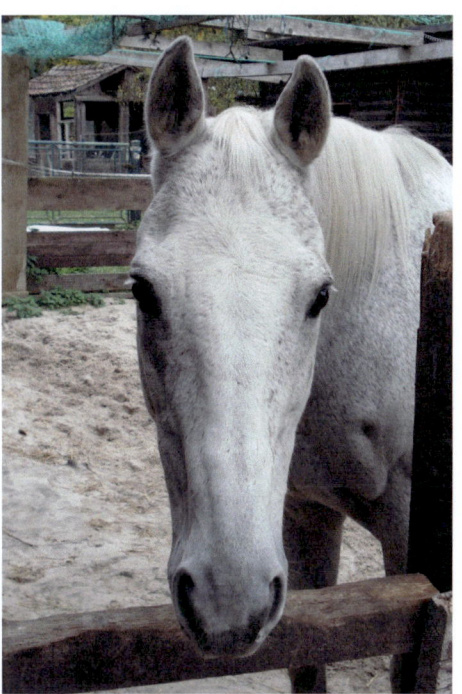

Horseradish can effectively fight a **wide range of bacterial infections**. I have not been able to study **viral infections** myself thoroughly. However, horseradish has certain **antiviral properties**, and I have indications that it is actually useful for such infections. Very high-dosed horseradish (about 50 grams per 100 kilograms of body weight) would be the drug of choice for me if a horse had a chronic or subacute form of Equine Infectious Anemia that is commonly considered incurable. The treatment is actually forbidden by law! (I think this is complete nonsense! How can a remedy then ever be found against it by the vets! By the pharmaceutical industry, one can hardly expect it, the disease is too rare and the profit expectations therefore too low!)

At least by no means does it harm to **give horseradish during a viral infection** additionally, because secondary infections by bacteria, which often pose a problem (often even the main problem!) with viral infections, are thereby quickly eliminated.

Observations show that for viral infections, during which horseradish was first given, and after that had shown no significant effect and antibiotics were then injected, the symptoms (e.g. edema of the legs and belly) even became worse, which had not happened with horseradish.

About at the same time as my investigations with horseradish with horses, similar experiments have been carried out on a substantially larger number of people (more than 1000!). In the **study** (Dr. U. Frank, Prof. Dr. K.F. Klippel), which did not use pure horseradish, but an **encapsulated dried combined preparation of horseradish and nasturtium** (a kind of cress), the effect on 13 clinically relevant kinds of bacteria which cause **infections** of the **urinary tract** and the **respiratory tract** were investigated. Like horseradish, **nasturtium** also generates **mustard oils** after destruction of its cell walls, however, these have a slightly different composition (for example it also generates benzyl mustard oil).

In this study, for the patients who took the nasturtium / horseradish drug the **same efficacy** was observed as in a control group which was treated with **synthetic antibiotics**! **Bactericidal action** and in lower dosage a **bacteriostatic effect** against **staphylococci**, **streptococci**, **enterococci**, **acinetobacter**, **E. coli**, **proteus**, **enterobacter** and **haemophili influenzae** was observed.

Moreover, there were also **virostatic effects** against **rhinovirus**, **influenza** and **Newcastle**. Besides, it showed **antimycotic effects** against **candida** and **mold fungi**.

The (German) over-the-counter medicine Angocin® used in the study contained 200 mg of dried nasturtium and 80 mg of dried horseradish per tablet, equivalent to about 2 grams of fresh herb and about 0.8 grams of fresh horseradish. However, according to manufacturer's data, the daily dosage for an adult is up to 25 tablets per day! This would then be equivalent to about 50 grams of fresh nasturtium and 20 grams of fresh horseradish if the manufacturing company should have managed to process the plants very gently.

However, I strongly suspect that much less of the fresh substances would be needed to achieve the same observed effect.

Information about the study can be found at

http://www.klinikum.uni-heidelberg.de/Phytomedizin-Traditionelles-Wissen-modern-genutzt.109013.0.html

The study expressly states that **formation of a resistance of germs is not to be expected**. In addition, it was found that the **active substances** are all already **resorbed in the small intestine**, so that the **bacterial flora in the large intestine is not damaged** as it would be with conventional antibiotics! If this is already an advantage for humans, then this applies even more to the "gut animal" horse! This might be the reason for their especially positive reaction towards horseradish!

The **study** on humans only considered **infections** which take place at locations at which the **main active substances** (mustard oils) of the horseradish and the nasturtium **concentrate** (**urinary** and **lung excretory pathways**). In my own investigations with horses I had also observed an **effect on other distant infected body parts** when horseradish was used in an about **two to three times higher dosage** (as compared to the locally effective dosage). For example it was effective in this higher dosage against phlegmons (streptococci) in the legs. Thus the active substances seem to be able to reach the sites of infections in sufficient amounts also via the bloodstream. The same is probably to be expected with humans.

Besides, in the **study** the **drug administration was evenly distributed throughout the day** which has turned out as less effective for horses according to my own investigations (except at very high dosages). In humans, it could therefore be similar. However, a more **even administration throughout the day** makes the intake, also of larger amounts, clearly **more pleasant and more tolerable**, particularly since people unlike horses do not eat it in hay-/grasscubes as an effective "diluting agent".

The encountered **virostatic** effect against influenza is very interesting!

According to this study, a **highly dosed intake of horseradish** (perhaps in combination with nasturtium) would be **recommendable** against **equine (and human!) influenza**! Maybe in this way some severity could be taken from a **deadly influenza wave** that scientists have been warning about for many years!

In October 2005 I have tested hints to a **virostatic effect** on myself (about 70 kilograms) when I suffered from an acute viral infection. According to this self-experiment, 25 grams of horseradish were still not sufficient for a distinct improvement. With 50 grams per day (about **70 grams per 100 kilograms of body weight**) a very distinct improvement in the state of health could be observed (on the next day). However, this amount is not pleasant to eat and already irritates the stomach. I had distributed the amount on 2 servings, one in the morning and one in the evening, because I think that, in contrast to the bactericidal effect, for the **virostatic effect** (the virus reproduction is only restrained) an about **constant amount of active substances in the body** is better. If the virus reproduction is sufficiently inhibited, the body's immune system gains time to effectively fight the virus.

During an influenza in autumn 2009 (probably swine influenza) I then tested on me the commercial medicine Angocin®. With 35 tablets a day (distributed on 5 times over the day) I took a clearly higher dosage than stated in the instructions for use, and thereby could kill off the influenza almost completely within 2 days. After 4 days I was completely healthy again. Besides, the intake was very tolerable!

The **ingestion of horseradish by people** is, according to my experience, most pleasant if you **cut the horseradish into several small pieces** (of several grams) and then **chew them one after the other in the mouth**, after (!) you have taken an **only small amount of cold milk** into the mouth **before chewing**. When **chewing the horseradish with little milk**, the very sharp gaseous mustard oils do not get into the windpipe or even the lung! Hence, during an outbreak of a **dangerous influenza epidemic** and lack of anti-viral drugs I would recommend the use of **horseradish** in humans as described, preferably in **combination with medicines which are good to the stomach**.

An **effect** of horseradish **against mold fungi** (as proven in the study with people) is supported by the case of my treatment of a big cart horse stallion which had an always recurring aspergilloma (a greenish stone-like mold fungus) in the paranasal sinus. After 2 months of feeding of 50 grams per 100 kilograms of body weight (400 grams per day distributed on 2 servings!) the aspergilloma did not come back again. The aspergilloma had been downright "burnt out".

During my experiments on the antibiotic use of horseradish, I came across the following scientific research, which I find so interesting that I would like to reproduce its content here, even though I did not test it myself, because I could successfully combat all infections with horseradish alone:

K. Allison et al. report in the renowned journal Nature (Vol. 473, 12.5.2011, p.216-220) that there is an easy way to effectively eliminate so-called "persisters" by a combination of antibiotics and the sugars glucose, fructose or mannitol! This also applied to bacteria in biofilms! Persisters are bacteria that have reduced their metabolism so far that antibiotics can no longer fight them because they are not absorbed into the bacteria. At a later stage, when no more antibiotics are present, persisters re-raise their metabolism and re-emerge. The sugar lures the persisters out of their state of rest, so to speak, and makes them vulnerable again!

Maybe it would also be possible to use horseradish, together with the described sugars, with success against persisters. So far, I have only used fructose together with ginger. There was also an, albeit slight, increase of its anti-inflammatory effect. I can not give a reason for this.

The following anecdote from history of science is, by the way, interesting and amusing: The **Count von Waldeck (1766-1875)** was a rather infamous than famous Maya researcher and had got around a lot in the world. He had, e.g., even been in Egypt with Napoleon. He reached an astonishing age of **109 years**, because, as he stated himself, he made a **6-week horseradish cure** every springtime! It is conceivable, that he reached this for our times biblical and for his times even astronomical age because the horseradish eliminated life-threatening infections already at the beginning.

Count von Waldeck is said to have have died, finally, of heart failure when he threw a glance on a young woman near the Champs Élysées!

Quick guide for feeding of horseradish to horses

Horseradish against bacterial infections

1.) **Quick increasing** of the dosage, beginning with about 20 grams in a meal, then 50 grams, 100 grams in a meal, ….. The horseradish should be **freshly grated** to achieve the best effectiveness.

Preferably, but not necessary for the antibiotic effect, the freshly grated horseradish is fed in **soaked hay-/grasscubes**. Particularly preferably together with a "well-being dosage" of **ginger** (1.5 to 2 grams per 100 kilograms of body weight), or even a higher dosage, if this is necessary (for inhibition of an inflammation).

Dosing target are **20 to 35 grams of horseradish per 100 kilograms of body weight**, depending on the severity of the infection. Even amounts of more than 50 grams per 100 kilograms of body weight have already been fed (in soaked hay-/grasscubes) in the case of borreliosis (Lyme disease) for several months. The borreliosis titer was thereby lowered to its normal range.

Horses, which are already used to horseradish can receive the full necessary amount immediately if this is required. The **antibiotic effect** (e.g. the decreasing of the swelling of a phlegmon) begins to set in **just after one day** when the required amount is reached and the wound is properly treated. (Otherwise, with constant new infections it is a fight against the tide!)

For treatment of **dental infections** (which are accessible from the mouth) and **coughing**, amounts of **10 to 12 grams per 100 kilograms of body weight** are usually sufficient. However, the gift of a higher dosage is also preferred here because by this means anti-bacterial substances are transported to the destination additionally via the bloodstream.

After a very (!) long-term administration of horseradish, an about 30% higher dosage should be given in case of a sudden onset of infectious diseases because in this case the effectiveness decreases a bit (presumably due to faster excretion of the active substances by the body).

2.) Maintaining the amount found for **at least 7 to 10 days** (as with conventional antibiotics too).

In foreseeable **long-term infections**, the amount should be kept **for several weeks** (from 4 to 8 weeks).

Borreliosis (Lyme disease) seems to require **especially high amounts** for an **even longer period of time**.

3.) In case of large dosages of horseradish the amount is reduced within several days.

4.) **For old horses** it is **in the long term recommended**:

Give an amount of **10 to 12 grams of freshly grated horseradish per 100 kilograms of body weight on two or three consecutive days a week** and every few months a daily dosage of 20 to 25 grams per 100 kilograms of body weight for about one week. **Even better**: in addition, **daily feed ginger** in an amount of 1.5 to 2 grams per 100 kilograms of body weight ("well-being dosage") or even more.

5.) For **emergencies** hold in stock a **large glass of preserved horseradish** (NOT the creamy version!) in your **medicine box at the stable**, which will give you time to give fresh horseradish the next day. However, preserved horseradish from the glass must be **dosed higher** (for safety's sake about **1.5 to 2 times higher**) because some of its ingredients are already partially degraded and the preserved horseradish is also diluted by other ingredients.

It is better to freeze horseradish for emergencies in larger pieces (about 50 grams) and to grate these frozen pieces when required and to feed the grated horseradish immediately. Also in this case, it must be fed about 1.5 times more, but such horseradish is better accepted by some horses than the preserved one from glasses! **People who feed their horses horseradish anyhow because of the teeth, best of all constantly keep in stock in the stable a triple dental dosage of fresh horseradish ready for use as an emergency dosage for other treatments.**

C. Licorice in horse feeding

Tests with 5 horses in 2009 over a period of up to 8 months have shown that it is possible to drastically reduce the symptoms of **headshaking** by feeding of **licorice** (the **plant** from which the sweet/candy is made). In the meantime, this has been confirmed for pollen-induced headshaking with more horses! In addition, a more exact investigation on my thoroughbred has shown that this feeding apparently also **fights the herpesvirus** which some doctors consider to be responsible for headshaking! Although there are not many reports from treated horses yet, I have decided to present the results as the effects on (pollen- and light-induced) headshaking occurred in each of the horses and were strong. (There was a so-called **strong causality or correlation**, respectively.) Owners of affected horses are thus enabled to help their 4-legged comrades at an early stage, which otherwise in some cases would even have to be euthanized for these reasons! And in cases of the dreaded and sometimes deadly **herpes epidemics**, in case of which veterinarians were so far powerless, licorice should, at least tentatively, be used in my opinion.

Not only in people are **allergies** on the rise since decades, but also in many animal species, including horses.
For riders particularly unpleasant is the so-called **headshaking**, because it greatly affects the use of the horse at certain times of the year.
The term headshaking for the disease describes the symptoms which occur especially during riding. In addition, the horses often try to rub the nose on the ground, on the wall or on the front legs to "wipe off" a permanent itch. The disease usually begins slightly and can increase to a degree that makes riding impossible. In extreme cases, the horses are so distracted that they endanger themselves, the rider and their surroundings. Often the **symptoms** occur only **seasonally**. Some headshakers are also **sensitive to light** (photosensitive) and sensitive to touch at the head.
In the past the blame was put simply on a too strong-acting rider's hand. Today we know that this can not always be the only explanation. If headshaking occurs only during certain seasons, it is obvious that **allergies**, e.g. to **pollen**, might be involved. The behavior can also be triggered by stress and in this case is comparable to the human burnout syndrome. **Stress** also causes an **increase** of an otherwise barely noticeable headshaking. Therefore, especially horses with a lot of thoroughbred in them are affected more often.
Mostly the treatment is very difficult, because the headshaking can be triggered by a number of causes and one often does not succeed in detecting the real one(s). Frequently there are also **several causes at the same time** involved in the triggering of the headshaking, each of which alone would not lead to it. (For example, also small "wolf teeth" in the jaw or an irritated hoof corium may worsen it.)
Some horses are **sensitive to light** (for those ones light-dampening headmasks are helpful). However, often **pollen** is the main cause of headshaking (similar to **hay fever**

in humans). An irritation is also recognizable by the fact that these animals constantly move the upper lip or/and sneeze frequently.

A close fitting **nasal net** does not eliminate the allergic reaction in such horses, which often rub their nose, because the coarse meshes cannot filter the pollen from the air. However, it brings relief to the horse, because it can rub its nose directly on the net.

An **irritation of the trigeminal nerve** is held responsible for the headshaking and rubbing of the nose. Some physicians also suspect an involvement of **latent ("sleeping") herpesviruses** in this nerve which are released by stress. (This is also my opinion on account of the investigations, which are later described.)

Veterinarians in many cases prescribe Cyroheptadin® which, however, is really satisfactory only in some cases and has, in addition, adverse side effects (apathy, risk of colic, inappetence). Other drugs are the anticonvulsants Carbamazepin® or Gabapentin® which are also prescribed for epilepsy.

Some horse owners also use the freely available antihistamines Loratadin® or Cetirizin®, but also without really satisfying effects. Besides, these cause fatigue as a side effect in the horse.

Surprisingly, it has now been shown since 2009 in experiments on several horses of different breeds that **licorice**, preferably in ground form, as a feed additive very effectively relieves headshaking of the horse (by about 90%)! This effect was noted in all observed horses. So there was a **strong causality/correlation** between the administration of licorice and the relief of the headshaking! And, very important: **Adverse side effects** were **not observed**!

An effect on other allergies, however, seems to be only weak. The underlying mechanism is unknown, but there seems to be involved a fight against the herpesvirus, which I would like to discuss later!

However, a component in licorice, **glycyrrhizin** (licorice sugar), has **strong side effects in humans at higher dosages**. It can affect the body's electrolyte balance, causing high blood pressure, headaches and edema. The reason is that glycyrrhizin influences the mineralcorticoid metabolism. (For this reason, the glycyrrhizin content in candy-licorice is generally reduced.)

Therefore, I was very careful in using **licorice** first, otherwise I would have tried it already 4 years earlier because it is supposed to have a **killing effect on herpesviruses** (which are also made responsible for headshaking). Moreover in Wikipedia (Germany) can be found (2013): „The sugar of licorice (glycyrrhizin) shall block the production of a virus protein of the herpesvirus which normally prevents the discovery of the virus by the cell. Without this protein, the cells notice the intruder and initiate their own death. However, the dosage required for this purpose is far too high to be reached by normal (harmless to health) consumption of licorice, and has not been proved in living humans, but only in cell cultures (J. Clin. Invest. 115 (3): 591-593 (2005).“

For the **contents of glycyrrhizin in licorice** different values are mentioned which range **between 3 and 14%** (according to different methods of analysis!). The time of harvest and the regional provenance are certainly crucial. But the method of analysis is certainly important for the determination of the true content!

The dosage found by me as necessary for a horse is depending on the strength of the symptoms, which depends on the type and amount of the triggering allergen (in the case of headshaking, e.g. the intensity of the flight of pollen), the inner excitement of the horse and the specific horse itself, and must be tested individually.

In general, for low allergen exposure, a decrease of the symptoms (e.g. nose rubbing) is already detectable for small quantities of about 1 gram of licorice per 100 kilograms of body weight. The effect then increases significantly with an increase of the dosage.

For headshakers reasonable dosages are between 1 and 10 grams per 100 kilograms of body weight, **usually around 5 grams per 100 kilograms of body weight**. However, these amounts are also dependent on the quality of the used licorice used, which naturally varies for natural products, and should be **tested individually**!

However, this is very simple, because you just slowly increase the amount until the desired effect has occurred.

But unlike ginger and horseradish, which have been safe to administer in all amounts observed so far, **more caution is needed with licorice**! Because of its mineralcorticoid effect, **high dosages** can lead to an **increase in the cortisol level** in the blood and at the same time to an **increase in the sodium level** and a **reduction in the potassium level**! This then leads to the formation of edemas, as is known as an undesirable adverse effect in humans in the case of giving cortisol. (Colloquially there is often spoken of cortison, however, it is always meant cortisol!) Although a change in the blood analysis data was noticeable for my English thoroughbred only for 8 grams per 100 kilograms of body weight after 1 ½ months of feeding this amount, whereby the values still were in the normal range and no edemas were noticeable, in my opinion at least **for higher dosages** (more than 5 grams per 100 kilograms of body weight) regular **controls of the blood analysis data by a veterinarian** should occur (period about all 2 months)!

For horses with metabolic disorders this should be done already with smaller amounts! The parameters to be supervised are the above mentioned **cortisol** (highly dependent on the time of day; thus it is necessary to always measure at about the same time of day to obtain reliable values!), **sodium** and **potassium**.

Generally it is advantageous to always adapt the dosage to the need and to lower the dosage accordingly when the allergy-triggering stimulus (e.g. the pollens in the late year) decreases. However, there are also good reasons not to fall below a certain dosage because the herpesviruses are still slowly killed by this amount if the allergen load has become quite low.

One should give licorice **not only over short periods of time as a cure**, **but permanently throughout the whole season during which headshaking occurs**, because in this way over time the **"pain memory"** of the horse is wiped out, which had "taught" its body to react already upon ever smaller quantities of allergen, to some extent even increased by excitement or panic.

The treatment of the horse should preferentially be started already some time before the desired alleviation of symptoms, and the **increasing of the dosage** should be done **slowly**, as should be usual for every change of feeding of horses.

As an example I report here about the successful treatment of my English thoroughbred, the first and best examined horse of the investigation. The other horses followed only later in spring and, hence, their **increasing of the dosage** occurred much faster (**within one to two weeks up to about 5 grams per 100 kilograms of body weight**).

My English thoroughbred (born in 1987) has been getting the licorice for more than 4 years during the pollen season. The interesting thing was that the **amount needed** for the same kind of alleviation of symptoms **decreased somewhat from year to year**. Particularly strong was this drop in the necessary dosage in the last year of observation (2012) before the new edition of the German version of this book. In this year only a maximum amount of licorice of just over 1.5 grams per 100 kilograms of body weight was needed and the horse nevertheless showed less symptoms than the year before! So there seems to be a kind of **partial healing** from the headshaking over the years! The reason for this is not clear yet.

Summary of the investigation on my English thoroughbred:

The investigation has been running for 4 years (2009 to 2012). By feeding licorice, the horse could be ridden again in the summer, and it also could enjoy the summer! From year to year, there was even further improvement that made it possible to lower the licorice dosages! Negative side effects did not occur at any of the dosages used. The **antibody titers** of equine herpesvirus-1 (EHV-1) and equine herpesvirus-4 (EHV-4) **significantly decreased in the first year** over the period of 8 months of feeding licorice by (at least) the factor 8 for EHV-1 and the factor 4 for EHV-4!

This had previously been thought impossible by my vet!

In the second year, the decrease of titers at the same dosage of licorice was noticeably lower, in the third year even lower and then almost disappeared in the fourth year! Although the titers were not in the range indicating an active disease at the beginning of feeding in 2009, it is important, in my opinion, that he treatment seems to offer the possibility to drive back the herpesvirus out of the nervous system even in the "dormant" (latent) state, something which had not been possible before and also was not even considered as possible!

It is surprising that the titers recovered during the period of non-feeding (winter), but the horse showed fewer symptoms at the same titer in the following year. But there exist so-called memory cells for antibodies in the body that provide antibodies in the long run even if there are no herpesviruses left anymore. In this respect, I still believe in the fighting of latent viruses by licorice and a reduction in the influence on the titer, the lower the amount of latent viruses in the nervous system becomes.

As a guideline, the required amounts **in the first year of treatment** were about 5 to 6 grams per 100 kilos of body weight. **In this investigation**, a medium-quality, but not old, **Chinese ground licorice** was used. (A presumably old batch from a tea shop had much less effect!)

The blood values were checked regularly.

Course of treatment of my horse:

English thoroughbred gelding, born 12.2.1987, 1.54 meters height, about 450 kilograms, in my possession since February 1994. Held in a large stall with large paddock. Fed with hay, grass, oats, apples, carrots; no mix-feeds or mineral supplements. Since September 2003 he receives ginger because of a keratoma in the right front hoof and melanoma at the root of the tail and since 2005 horseradish three times a week, to maintain the health of the dental apparatus.

At least one comprehensive blood analysis has been made each year since the start of the feeding of ginger to the horse. Ginger and horseradish had no obvious, observable effects on the usually measured parameters of the comprehensive blood analysis which could be compared with previous sporadically blood tests. (But ginger had a strong lowering effect on the seldom measured cortisol!)

The horse had been a headshaker since its purchase in February 1994, however, the headshaking had increased over the years. Deterioration episodes were caused by herpes vaccinations with active and passive vaccine in 2001 and by an unsuccessful desensitization against pollen; an improvement had occurred, however, by omitting of supplements and of feed containing supplements that he had received for several years until the year 2000. There was also a clear correlation between the degree of irritation in the right front hoof caused by a keratoma and the extent of headshaking.

In 2009, an attempt to decrease the headshaking during the time of flying pollen by feeding of licorice was started on account of the hypothesis that herpes could be involved in headshaking.

The following listing shows the timetable of the fed licorice amounts and the relevant blood values. Apart from sodium and potassium, cortisol was also checked, as well as the antibody titers of EHV-1 and EHV-4.

For daily quantities higher than 2 grams per 100 kilograms of body weight the licorice was distributed evenly into the morning and evening feed. The sampling for the blood analyses took place (converted to the standard wintertime) between 18:15 and 19:00, in each case in a range between 15 and 60 minutes after the administration of the concentrated feed which included the evening dose of licorice. Throughout the investigation (and long before!), the horse received 4 grams, in the last two years, 5 grams of granulated Nigerian ginger per 100 kilograms of body weight in its evening feed. The evening licorice administration took place together with the ginger in soaked (not dripping) fiber-rich hay-/grasscubes (about 0.5 kilograms of dry matter plus water). The morning administration of licorice occurred in rolled oats which were only slightly moistened with very little water, so that the licorice powder adhered to it and could not get into the nostrils of the horse by breathing.

Increases of the licorice dosage took place to compensate for an increasing pollen load. Reduction of the amount took place when the pollen load (and with it the headshaking) apparently decreased.

However, in October of the first year the amount was not further reduced, although the pollen load had decreased sharply. The reason was to be able to examine the influence of licorice on the herpes titers at low pollen load.

From 26.2.2009:   daily 0.5 gram of licorice per 100 kilograms of body weight
from 4.3.2009:   daily 1 gram of licorice per 100 kilograms of body weight
from 8.3.2009:   daily 1.5 grams of licorice per 100 kilograms of body weight
from 3.4.2009:   daily 2 grams of licorice per 100 kilograms of body weight
from 11.4.2009:   daily 2.5 grams of licorice per 100 kilograms of body weight
On 15.4.2009 blood analysis:
Cortisol: 2.0 micrograms / deciliter (standard value: 2,9-9,1)
EHV-1 antibody titer: 1:64 (standard value: ≤1:64)
EHV-4 antibody titer: 1:128 (standard value: ≤1:256)
Sodium: 142 millimoles/liter (standard value: 125-150)
Potassium: 4.5 millimoles/liter (standard value: 2,8-4,5)
Values for EHV-1 of 1:64 and EHV-4 of 1:128 had already been found in 2004 at the end of July. 2 weeks earlier they had been 1:64 and 1:64, respectively.

From 20.4.2009:   daily 3 grams of licorice per 100 kilograms of body weight
from 26.4.2009:   daily 4 grams of licorice per 100 kilograms of body weight
from 1.5.2009:   daily 4.5 grams of licorice per 100 kilograms of body weight
from 9.5.2009:   daily 5.5 grams of licorice per 100 kilograms of body weight
On 19.5.2009 blood analysis:
Cortisol: 1.9 micrograms / deciliter (standard value: 2,9-9,1)
EHV-1 antibody titer: 1:12 (standard value: ≤1:64)
EHV-4 antibody titer: 1:64 (standard value: ≤1:256)
Sodium: 140 millimol/liter (standard value: 125-150)
Potassium: 4.2 millimol/liter (standard value: 2,8-4,5)
My veterinarian had been very much surprised about this result of the blood analysis and remarked that she could not imagine another decrease of the herpes titers below the value of 1:12.

From 22.5.2009:   daily 6 grams of licorice per 100 kilograms of body weight
from 5.6.2009:   daily 7 grams of licorice per 100 kilograms of body weight
from 8.6.2009:   daily 8.5 grams of licorice per 100 kilograms of body weight
On 16.7.2009 blood analysis:
Cortisol: 7.8 micrograms / deciliter (standard value: 2,9-9,1)
EHV-1 antibody titer: 1:16 (standard value: ≤1:64)
EHV-4 antibody titer: 1:64 (standard value: ≤1:256)
Sodium: 144 millimol/liter (standard value: 125-150)
Potassium: 3.2 millimol/liter (standard value: 2,8-4,5)

The EHV-1 value had risen a bit again what might be linked, however, to the very high pollen load at this time, due to which a higher licorice amount was given which, however, apparently was not completely sufficient to fight all released herpesviruses.

Symptomatically the headshaking had also increased a bit in spite of the raised dosage as compared to the previous investigation. This showed that a further increase of the licorice dosage would have in fact been necessary, which was not carried out, however, because of uncertainty about eventual adverse health effects, even if no edemas had been observed.

This time the value for cortisol was clearly heightened compared to the previous investigation, but still within the standard range. The potassium value started to decline, but was also still within standard range.

After this blood analysis, the licorice dosage was lowered because the peak of the pollen load was apparently exceeded.

From 16.7.2009:   daily 6 grams of licorice per 100 kilograms of body weight
from 18.7.2009:   daily 5.5 grams of licorice per 100 kilograms of body weight
On 28.10.2009 blood analysis:
Cortisol: 1.5 micrograms / deciliter (standard value: 2,9-9,1)
EHV-1 anti-body titer: 1:6 (standard value: ≤1:64)
EHV-4 anti-body titer: 1:32 (standard value: ≤1:256)
Sodium: 141 Millimol/liter (standard value: 125-150)
Potassium: 4.0 Millimol/liter (standard value: 2,8-4,5)

Without a high load of pollen the diminished amount of licorice had at the end of October managed to decrease the herpes titer for EHV-1 as well as for EHV-4.

The effect of licorice on EHV-1 seems to be stronger than that on EHV-4. The effect on other herpesvirus types was not examined. However, an effect is likely, because the types are related to each other.

In 2010, the same procedure was followed, but the feeding of licorice in low dosage already started in mid-January when there were no symptoms yet. (Blood analyses were conducted on January 13th, April 15th, July 8th, August 5th, October 28th, and November 24th.) Until April, the dosage was then increased to about 5.5 grams per 100 kg body weight, and from June up to about 6 grams per 100 kilos of body weight. From the beginning of October, the dosage was then reduced to 4 grams per 100 kilograms of body weight and in early November further reduced within a week.

Even without licorice feeding, the EHV-1 titer started with only 1: 8 in January and dropped to 1: 6 during the maximum licorice dosing. At the end of the year, however, after the completion of the licorice feeding, it was again at 1:24. The EHV-4 titer started at 1:32 in January and then slowly increased to 1:64 during the year.

Despite the increase in EHV titers as compared to the previous year, less headshaking was shown, although the dose was slightly reduced compared to the previous year. The cortisol level only once in July reached a value of 3.5 micrograms per deciliter and was otherwise at 2.0 to 2.4, certainly due to the simultaneous feeding of ginger.

In 2011, the procedure was essentially the same as in 2010, with the same dosages. Blood analyses were carried out on 14.1., 16.3., 17.5., 11.8. and 9.11.. Again, the horse reacted less to pollen than the year before. Hence, there had been another, if not strong, improvement. This improvement also showed in spite of EHV titers, which from the beginning of the year were significantly higher than in the previous year. At the beginning of 2011, the EHV-1 titer was 1:32 and the EHV-4 titer was 1:64. In August, the EHV-1 was 1:18 and the EHV-4 1:64. And in November, with no pollen activity and no licorice feeding, the EHV-1 was 1:64 and the EHV-4 was 1:32. The maximum cortisol value was 3.8 micrograms per deciliter in August, otherwise 2.1 to 2.7.

In the year 2012, the licorice feeding started much later (beginning of March), as symptoms started to appear very late! In addition, only a significantly (!) lower maximum amount of licorice (only 1.5 grams per 100 kilograms of body weight) was needed than the years before and at the same time with significantly less symptoms as reaction on pollen load! Apparently, a partial healing of the pollen allergy had occurred during the winter. But the reasons are not clear.
Blood analyses were carried out on 21.2., 15.5., 5.8 and 15.11. The EHV-1 titer was 1:64 in February and 1:32 in May. The EHV-4 titer was 1:32, then 1:48 in May. In August, the EHV titers were accidentally not investigated. Both values were 1:32 in November. The cortisol levels peaked at 4.8 micrograms per deciliter in May, otherwise they were 1.4 (two times) to 2.1. The low values of 1.4 were measured when the horse was given a ginger dose of 15 grams per 100 kilograms of body weight and at the same time 25 grams of freshly grated horseradish per 100 kilograms of body weight due to an illness in August, and after the five-week horseradish treatment of his teeth suppuration in October 2012 (see part B of the book).

Surprisingly, it has thus been found in the long-lasting (over almost 4 years) experiment to treat headshaking that it is possible to give **horses** therapeutically **sufficient dosages** of licorice **in the long term** without side effects. The horses also showed much more joy at work and were looking forward to leave the stable area and be able to train! They also seemed to sweat less.
The treatment also seems to **lower** the **herpes titers** very clearly in the beginning. In my opinion, this is only possible because even "dormant" viruses in the nervous system are destroyed. Why the titer rises again in later years without a resurgence of symptoms is unclear. However, so-called memory cells of the immune system could play a role here.

Surprisingly, the **level of cortisol** in the blood of my thoroughbred was **lower** in most cases **than the standard range**. This is presumably due to the long-term feeding of ginger. In spite of his 25 years (2012) the value of cortisol corresponded instead to that of a **very young horse**! Only at the time of the feeding of the maximum amount of licorice did it get into the standard range for his age group. (Also in humans, the standard range of cortisol levels in the blood increases with age.)
Although a value for cortisol from the time before the investigation of treatment of headshaking by licorice is not known (cortisol does not belong to the usual values of a blood analysis), a decreasing of the cortisol value in the blood by the feeding of ginger

casually explains, why **ginger helps** horses who, e.g., suffer from **Equine Cushing Syndrome** (ECS)!

(This effect was seen as a positive side effect in Cushing horses with arthrosis which were treated with ginger for their arthroses.) Cushing horses show among other things an excess of cortisol in their blood which leads to the symptoms typical of the illness (e.g. delayed change of coat, etc.). **Horses** that receive **ginger**, however, change their coat more easily and also look **younger** in general!

The somewhat lower than standard value of cortisol obviously does not have negative side effects. Presumably this is even advantageous! I suppose, it is the reaction of the body to the fact that by the feeding of ginger there already exist enough anti-inflammatory substances in the body. The lower value of cortisol also explains, why the immune system is not affected by ginger, although anti-inflammatory substances generally weaken it. (Cortisol weakens the immune system against germs!)

All this suggests that it is possible to reduce the level of cortisol in the blood by feeding of ginger and thereby counteract possible adverse effects of the licorice at high dosages. Reasonable dosages are about 4 grams of ginger per 100 kilograms of body weight which can be reached by slowly increasing its amount within about one week.

However, since no edemas or other symptoms of a too high level of cortisol in the blood occurred with the 4 other horses of the 2009 experiment (no negative side effects could be registered generally!), dosages up to 6 grams of licorice per 100 kilograms of body weight which were administered to these horses, seem still to be safe even without feeding of ginger.

To be reliable, blood analyses for determining the content of cortisol in the blood always have to be taken at about the same time of the day, because the cortisol level depends very much on the time of day! Otherwise there is no reliable value at hand to decide, whether the value of cortisol begins to change strongly. The supervising veterinarian should thus make his visit at the right time of the day! (In humans the value of cortisol drops at night and increases in the morning again. For horses this is probably similar.)

About the mode of action of licorice one can only speculate, because more detailed investigations are still missing. In my opinion, it is a combination of at least two **modes of action**, an **antiallergic** and an **antiviral** against the herpesvirus.

(Licorice might also have an antiviral effect against another virus, eventually involved in headshaking. Bornaviruses are also in the discussion from time to time. Licorice acts not only specifically against the herpesvirus, but also against other viruses. In Japan, licorice sugar (glycyrrhizin) is used, for example, in case of chronic hepatitis C.)

That licorice is already efficient in relatively small quantities and, moreover, acting very quickly (within one day) at low pollen concentrations, points also to an anti-allergic action.

An anti-viral action is in my opinion strongly supported by the fact that even after cessation of licorice feeding the headshaking remained clearly diminished in situations in which the horse otherwise would have shaken its head badly even without pollen flight, e.g. in rain or fog. Apparently, a partial healing of the headshaking has taken place during the feeding of licorice! This could be explained elegantly by a decrease of the amount of latent viruses in the trigeminal nerve during the course of the licorice treatment.

In addition to the supposed anti-allergic and the (in humans) proven antiviral effect, also **another mechanism of action is possible**: Among many other substances, licorice contains also **isoliquiritigenin**, a substance that can block or reduce the production of the neurotransmitter dopamin in the nervous system. This should lead to a reduction of pain or itch transmission in the nervous system!
However, presumably it is a **sum of several effects by different components** (also other, not examined ones) **in licorice** which leads to a clearly observable overall effect.

Research about the exact mechanisms of action at universities would be desirable and could lead to further optimizations, also for people!

Quick guide for feeding of licorice to horses

Licorice against headshaking or to fight herpes

1.) **Slowly increase** the amount up to about **5 to 6 grams per 100 kilograms of body weight within about one to two weeks**. The licorice is preferably ground or like semolina and should not be too old. The wholesale trade presumably has more suitable licorice than tea houses because their product is more fresh.
Licorice is well accepted by most horses. It is fed preferentially in soaked hay-/grasscubes or in slightly moistened concentrate feed (e.g. rolled oats), so that the powder is not inhaled into the nostrils. (Very unpleasant!)
Preferably the daily amount is distributed into the **morning and the evening feed**. The feed for the morning feeding can already be prepared on the day before, by moistening the concentrate with very little water (usually one full palm is enough) and then adding the licorice and distributing it by stirring. Although the water is soaked up or evaporated until the morning, the powder still sticks to the surface of the concentrate and does not form dust which might get inhaled into the nostrils of the horse. Moreover, by doing so the feed does not stick to the bucket while emptying it. Before starting to feed licorice, it makes sense in my opinion to have a **blood analysis** made that includes **cortisol**, **sodium** and **potassium**. (The **equine herpes titers** are **optional** (unfortunately not cheap); anyway, they are interesting.) Then you know from which blood values you started.

2.) If the dosage of licorice is sufficient (significant decrease in headshaking), you maintain this dosage. About one month after reaching the dosage you have a blood analysis made. If the dosage is not sufficient, the licorice amount is further increased. **Higher dosages** should be particularly **supervised for the occurrence of symptoms**, e.g. edemas. In the case of dosages of more than 6 grams per 100 kilograms of body weight, a controlling blood analysis should in my opinion be made every two months. In case of a dosage of 5 to 6 grams per 100 kilograms of body weight, a controlling blood analysis is probably sufficient every three months and a significant change in the blood values is not to be expected then, except if the horse should be handicapped in its health.

3.) After the end of the headshaking season (often the end of the pollen flight), the dosage of licorice is **decreased within about one week**. A control blood analysis before the end of feeding licorice is interesting.

D. Treatment of fungal skin diseases of horses

Fungal skin diseases (cutaneous mycosis) of horses are often **tediously** to treat with the classical drugs which are prescribed by the veterinarian and they often reoccur by **re-infection** over and over again, especially in riding schools in which the same cleaning equipment or the same saddles are used for different horses.

By a short scientific communication of the **Botanical Institute of the University of Bonn (Prof. Frahm)** I was made aware of the **extremely strong fungicidal (antimycotic) effect of mosses**. It was also pointed out in this short article that the alcoholic extract of some mosses even acts **significantly more fungicidal than commercially available fungicides** for the treatment of plants (and humans) with fungal infections.

I tested this for the first time when two of the horses in our stable got a fungal skin infection at several places (bare skin) of their tail roots. In case of the appearance of such a fungal skin infection I had previously and with success used a chemical product with the active substance econazol. With just two to three treatments with this substance I had always been able to eliminate this fungal infections at the tail root.

But in the two new cases I had (instead of econazol) simply applied and rubbed a slightly moistened mud of **mashed moss**, which just happened to grow in front of the box door, onto the affected areas. Already this one treatment was enough to completely delete the fungal infetion on both affected horses in all places! The grated moss had proved to be more effective than a strong commercially available antimycotic drug! (A former classmate has even freed a goldfish with grated moss from a fungal infection, and later, with a very diluted moss extract, a catfish.)

Curious about these quick healings, I tried to find out a bit more about the reasons for this phenomenal effectiveness (which also works for fungal infections of skin and nails of **humans**! Mosses are also very effective in the case of **lichens**, since these are a symbiosis of fungus and algae!)

An explanation can be found in the **origin of the mosses**: Mosses exist since **hundreds of millions of years**. In this long time they lived in a **humid environment** in which they had to defend themselves constantly against fungal infections. In this lasting defense they have forged a whole cocktail of active substances into a shield that no fungus could break and this, although mosses frequently even grow side by side with mushrooms. But any fungal spore that happens to falls on the moss, is killed by its active substances that sit in the cell walls.

I also had the type of moss I used first determined (by Prof. Frahm), and it was mainly bryum argenteum with small admixtures of ceratodon purpureus, both so-called **bryophyta** which even belong to the mosses with the least fungicidal effect and are widespread. So-called **liverworts** are **most effective**. However, for some of them of which some grow at trees (not to be mistaken with lichens!), allergic skin reactions are known after a long lasting contact. With the frequent bryophyta mosses this is not to be expected, since lying on a mossy meadow would otherwise already have become fatal for many people. The body has already adapted well to the contact with these plants.

The **Native Americans of North America** use crushed **moss** even for **wound treatment**, as it also has an **antibacterial effect**. This bactericidal effect had also already been used by the **Vikings**: On their journeys they had their fish wrapped in **peat moss**. Successful trials have also been carried out at the University of Trondheim. The fish was then preserved for weeks, however, it acquired a dark color, needing getting used to!

Prof. Frahm has even drunk moss extract (produced with white wine), and it has apparently been good for him, as he reported. And in the stomach of the glacier mummy "Ötzi" unusually large amounts of moss were found. This is an indication that the healing effects of mosses were already known to humans 5,000 years ago.

When applying **self-harvested moss**, care must only be taken that the moss is **not harvested during frost**! Strangely enough such moss has hardly any fungicidal properties any more! Otherwise, even from a one year old dried moss an alcoholic, highly effective extract can be obtained.

Especially for the treatment of a fungal infection which sits deep in and under a **fur coat**, **alcoholic extracts are better suited** than mush of mashed moss because they are of **low viscosity** and thereby get deep into the fur. In **Germany** one can buy **alcoholic liverwort extract** ("Lebermooser"), e.g. via a chemist's shop, or through the internet (www.niem-handel.de). It has already proven itself in the meantime with many hundred horses. A friend also uses it to successfully treat foot fungus in a nursing home.

The pharmaceutical industry had of course also become attentive to the strong fungicidal effect. However, the research, despite proven efficacy, was completely stopped after it was found out that not a single, definite extractable substance was responsible for the effect, but the combined effect of a complicated mixture of many active substances. As soon as they began to separate the extremely effective extract, the individual fractions showed less and less effectiveness! Thus no sound basis for patenting, the basis for later profits, was possible anymore and, moreover, a drug approval extremely difficult.

The case of the mosses shows by way of example, how good research can be prevented by exclusively commercial considerations! But (with constantly rising health insurance costs!) it must not be, that effective treatments are not used just because there is nothing to be earned with them, or because their otherwise proven effect cannot be explained (up to now) due to their complexity!

In summary, by treating with mosses or moss extracts **all or at least most fungal skin infections or lichens** on horses (and people!) can be treated well and **without side effects**.

In addition to the treatment of fungi with mosses or moss extract, I would like to point out that some **fungal skin infections** on humans are **strongly favored by consumption of sugar** and can sometimes, despite medication, only be eliminated if the **consumption of sugar is strongly reduced** for some time! This certainly also applies to horses! Hence, in case of frequent returns of fungal skin infections, the (anyhow doubtful) feeding of molasses (molasses-containing mueslis!) but also of other feed with easily digestible carbohydrates, should be stopped. Ideally you only give hay, or hay and some oats.

Another use of liverwort extract, in combination with cod liver oil, to inhibit growth of equine sarcoids, is discussed in Chapter H.

Quick guide to treatment of fungal skin infections:

a.) **Mashing of moss together with very little water** and daily **application of the pulp** on the affected skin. At the latest after about three days bare skin should be free from the fungus!
Or (preferred):

b.) Use of **commercially available alcoholic liverworts extract**. **Dilute with water at a ratio of 1:5 to 1:10** and **apply to the skin or rub into the coat thoroughly** to ensure that all fungal spores are reached. (Attention: The direction of use of a dilution 1:200, which is indicated on the bottle, applies only to plants and only as a prophylaxis! **For fungal diseases of the skin, this is not enough!** An indication for use against fungal skin infections was omitted because of a **claim for damages by the pharmaceutical industry!**) Also in this case the fungus is usually already killed after the first treatment, but for safety's sake the treatment should be continued for some time, particularly as fungal spores hide in the fur or skin fat.

E. Ambulant treatment of keratomas

Keratomas are excrescenses of bad quality horn at the inner surface of the hoof wall which can exert pressure onto the hoof corium and thus lead to lameness. The cause for their formation is not really clear, probably there is not just one possible cause. Pussy hoof abscesses, which find their way up the hoof wall and leak through the coronet can be mentioned here, but also other injuries at the coronet, which lead to growing down of faulty horn structures.

Keratomas are a constant danger for the formation of **pussy hoof abscesses**, because along the inferior horn of the keratoma germs can penetrate unmolested up to the hoof corium and lead to infections there. (Hence, frequent abscesses at the same place of the same hoof strongly point to the existence of a keratoma!) Moreover, often a **channel** forms along or in the keratoma in the direction of the hoof corium, because the keratoma irritates the corium and the forming **inflammatory liquid** looks for a way outside which most easily leads through the inferior horn of the keratoma.

In the long run, keratomas lead to a **regression of the coffin bone** which lies behind the hoof corium onto which the keratoma exerts pressure. This regression of the bone by the pressure of the keratoma is clearly visible on X-ray pictures. If the coffin bone gets too thin in this region, it can even break!

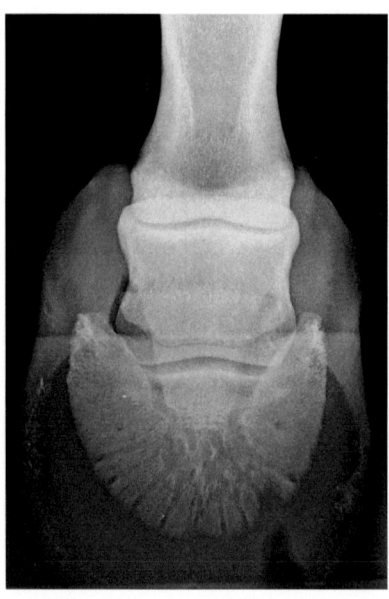

This picture of April 2008 shows the coffin bone of my thoroughbred, which is damaged by the keratoma in his right front hoof. The keratoma, and with it the notch in the coffin bone, had become ever larger over the years.

One can also recognize where sole horn was removed to release pressure onto the keratoma. By this measure the lameness disappeared because the forces of the keratoma onto the corium decreased.

The classical treatment of keratomas is the **opening of the hoof wall** under anesthesia (if necessary up to the coronet) and the **removal of the entire keratoma**! The hoof is weakened very much by this procedure and up to the time, when the hoof wall has grown down far enough again, a use of the horse is only very limited, if possible at all. By load removal from the operated hoof and due to the long healing time, there can also originate secondary damages in other limbs or malpositions in the back.

An alternative treatment is to try to adapt the loads in the hoof by **hoof-orthopedic measures** in such a way that the **keratoma gets smaller with time** and **grows out** by itself. By this procedure the keratoma is thus not removed surgically.

However, this second procedure is also not always applicable. The keratoma in the hoof further exerts pressure onto the corium, and hence the horse does not load its hoof correctly. And if the faulty horn of the keratoma is forming all the time because of an injury at the coronet, it can never grow out!

For my English thoroughbred with a thin hoof wall and sole, the following method of treatment, which represents a middle course between the classical and the alternative method of treatment, has proved promising after a long time of experimenting.

1.) The hoof is brought into a correct form in the **hoof-orthopedic sense**.

2.) The **keratoma** is first cut out with a hoof knife as far as possible **from the sole upwards**, and then the **keratoma is further scraped out upwards** with a so-called „**sharp curette**" (bone curette) of the smallest or second-smallest size (as the veterinarians uses it, e.g. for scraping out in the jaw bone), without destroying the hoof wall itself. Best of all you scrape the way upwards along the channel in or along the keratoma until no more channel can be seen. In this way you create a **defined opening** that can be kept clean. The resulting cavity is best shaped so that one or more small pieces of cotton wool, which are pressed into it later, do not fall out ("blind hole").

3.) The cavity is then preferably filled with a **mild disinfectant**, which does not harm hoof horn. Microdacyn® (formerly Dermacyn®) has proven particularly suitable for this purpose. Microdacyn® is an aqueous solution of compounds which contain oxygen and chlorine (it smells like a swimming pool after a busy day!) and has also proven to be effective in the treatment of difficult-to-heal skin injuries of humans. It is innocuous (even in the eye!), and it can also be used at the horse very well for many purposes of wound disinfection! Since it also contains gaseous disinfecting compounds, it penetrates deep into horny crevices, but obviously does not harm the horn.

4.) Afterwards you stuff clean **cotton wool** into the cavity which is still filled with the disinfectant and press the cotton together tightly. (Alternatively, you can of course stuff soaked cotton into the hole.) In case of a suitably shaped cavity it will not fall out later. The stuffed cotton is still compressible and, hence, does not exert pressure onto the corium as a keratoma does.

5.) Finally, you can additionally glue an **adhesive tape** across the opening to be on the safe side. For this purpose I use protective tapes (of good quality) as they are used by painters. Though these tapes are destroyed fast, until this happens the cotton in the cavity is further compressed by the movement of the horse.

6.) The cotton wool plug should be changed **every one to 2 days** and the cavity thereby cleaned again with the sharp curette. This happens best in the evening in the stable. Since the hoof wall is abraded at the bottom and grows down from above, the **cavity**

must be reshaped about once a week with the sharp curette. If you fail to do this, after a while the horse will start to put more uneven weight on this hoof, when it feels more pressure by the keratoma onto the corium again.

By this method I have completely prevented the development of abscesses in the hoof of my bare-hoof horse with very sensitive hoofs, and additionally the hoof as a whole began to grow down more correctly from the top for the first time. However, the notch in the coffin bone still persists with this measure. An X-ray examination 1 ½ years after the begin of the treatment showed no improvement in the coffin bone, but also no deterioration!

Another and very(!) clear improvement in the treatment of keratomas coincidently resulted from the treatment of a horny cleft (sandcrack), which had originated in the middle of the toe, because the horse now loaded the hoof more centrally after the afore described treatment. The cleft was formed at the site of the indentation of the coffin bone (so-called "crena marginis solearis") in the middle of the front of the hoof, which is recognizable as a small indentation in the above X-ray image. Since the new correct load was now unusual for the hoof, the crena acted as a predetermined breaking point.

After the horny cleft continued to move upwards and could not be controlled by the previous hoof processing, the gap was bridged by means of a **resin-bound glass fiber fabric**, as described in the following **chapter F, "Treatment of cracks in hooves"**.

Surprisingly at first glance, this **glued-on fiberglass-bridge made the keratoma distinctly more resilient!** In retrospect, however, there is a very simple and logical explanation for this: The **fiberglass-bridge thickened the hoof wall** above the keratoma, and this thickening of the wall makes the **wall less deformable by the hoof mechanism**. But if the hoof wall is less deformed, then the **keratoma also presses less** against the corium! As a result, the corium is not inflamed so much any more, and less or even no inflammatory liquid is produced. At my horse this was observable by the decrease of the size of the channel which had always formed along the keratoma down to the white line.

However, the glued-on fiberglass-bridge and the positive effect resulting from it, still show something else: **At a hoof with a keratoma, hoof orthopedists should not rasp thin the hoof wall at its lower half** to control and regulate the abrasion of the horn! Instead the hoof walls should be **rasped thin only at the lower edge or not at all**, so that the thickness of the hoof wall is preserved as much as possible! As physics teaches us, a thinning of the hoof wall has a dramatic effect on its flexibility: The reason is that the **force** which is necessary for deforming the hoof wall follows an **equation** in which the **thickness of the hoof wall enters with the third power!** In other words, by **halving the thickness** of the hoof wall, this can then be bent already **with only an eighth of the force** that would be necessary for a normal hoof wall thickness! Although the hoof is not thinned out across the whole area of the wall and also the internal structures of the hoof stabilize it, nevertheless, the effect is very strong! If the hoof wall is weakened, then the coffin bone, which is already endangered in case of a keratoma, is more heavily loaded!

Hence: At hoofs with keratomas the hoof wall must not be rasped thinner! The correction of the abrasion must be done in the lowest part of the hoof ("mustang role") and must be done much more often!

It was interesting to see whether the glued-on glassfiber-bridge on the hoof wall which I had glued on further on, even after the sandcrack had grown down, would cause the keratoma to grow out over time, because the fiberglass-bridge thickened the wall beyond the natural thickness, thereby decreasing its flexibility. Thus, the thicker wall compensated for the lack of stability of the notched coffin bone and thus normalized the flexibility of the hoof as a whole.

From a phenomenological point of view, the hoof then behaves more like a normal hoof! (A classical horseshoe also restricts the movement of the horn capsule. However, it does so not physiologically, but very unevenly only at the lower edge. There are then concentrations of the forces on the nails, whereas the gluing on the hoof wall is very uniform, just as if the horse has a thicker hoof wall.)

However, I have **not been able to observe a growing out of the keratoma** in my thoroughbred. But there was **no deterioration**. For other horses, however, the procedure described may still be helpful for a growing out, because of course, it depends very much on the cause of the keratoma!

As already remarked in the foreword for this English edition, **I now very much recommend the use of the relatively new F-balance-method** (www.f-balance.com) for the preparation of hoofs! It is **also recommendable for hoofs with keratoma**, because it gives the structures of the hoof just those loads which they want to get! And a keratoma does not like to get much load!

F. Treatment of cracks in hooves (sandcracks)

Sandcracks are often caused by permanent incorrect loading of the hoof, e.g. by a **wrong form of the hoof relative to the limbs**. However, they can also occur at **weak spots** of the hoof ("scar horn") or as a result of generally **bad hoof horn** or due to **bad horse-shoeing**. In many cases, sandcracks can be eliminated by **correct hoofcare** and then simply grow out. Things are different in case of structural weaknesses of the hoof or if the capsule of the hoof is very often loaded unilaterally because of **stony, uneven ground**. Then cracks, once formed, can hardly grow out, because the long lever arm with each one-sided load transmits strong forces to the origin of the crack by which the horn at this point is torn over and over again.

In the case of my thoroughbred, the sandcrack originated in the exact middle of the toe, after a hoofcare procedure (see chapter E) had let him put more load on his keratoma again and thus he rolled his hoof again more centrally over his toe. After the sandcrack did not make any attempt to grow out despite proper hoofcare, I decided to **bridge** the **crack** in a simple manner and to thereby prevent the transmission of forces to the origin of the crack to allow it to grow down.

The state-of-the-art procedure for this are steel bands that span the crack and are affixed with screws in the hoof wall. However, this treatment seemed to me less favorable because thereby the spreading forces acting onto the crack are concentrated only at the screws in the horn. Therefore, I have **bridged the crack by fiberglass-reinforced plastic** which was polymerized onto the hoof wall.

Particularly **fiberglass fabric** (instead of fiberglass fleece) is suited for this because the fabric can **transmit strong forces unidirectionally**, if it adheres with the fibers perpendicular to the crack.

As a plastic that fills the fabric and connects to the horn, **acrylic resins**, **epoxy resins** and, more recently, **polyurethanes** are commercially available, the latter two especially for use on horse hooves.

I myself have worked with epoxy resin as well as with acrylic resin and I favor the simple **acrylic resin**, which can be bought cheaply, as well as as the fiberglass fabric, as a **repair kit for boathulls and cars** in do-it-yourself stores. (The treatment of the sandcrack of my thoroughbred, until it had grown out after half a year, had cost me only about 6 euros/dollars of material!) Although epoxy resins are of higher quality than acrylic resins and additionally more resistant to water, they are also more viscous and worse to work with. Since the resin does not have to hold a shoe on the hoof, the acrylic resin, which is only one component mixed with a hardener, is completely sufficient.

Nevertheless epoxy resins are very useful and necessary in cases in which a stronger gluing is needed or a thicker layer must be put onto the hoof.

The following pictures demonstrate the course of the treatment of the sandcrack of my thoroughbred. Unfortunately, the pictures do not start when the sandcrack had its maximum length and extended over half of the toe wall because I did not know at that time if it would work at all. The first application (with epoxy resin) had already taken place in mid-June 2009 and had lasted for 5 weeks.

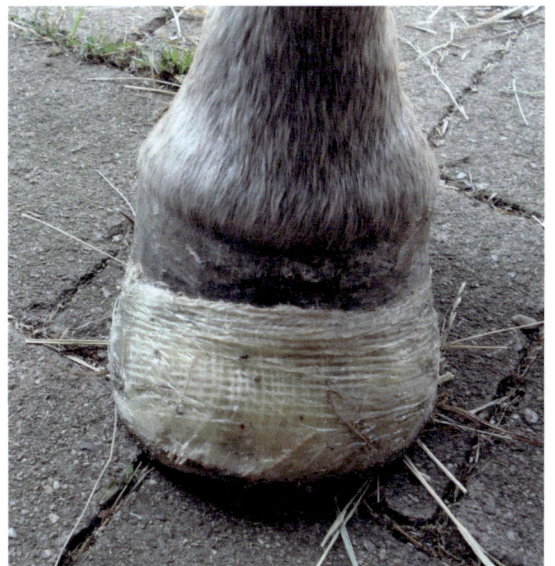

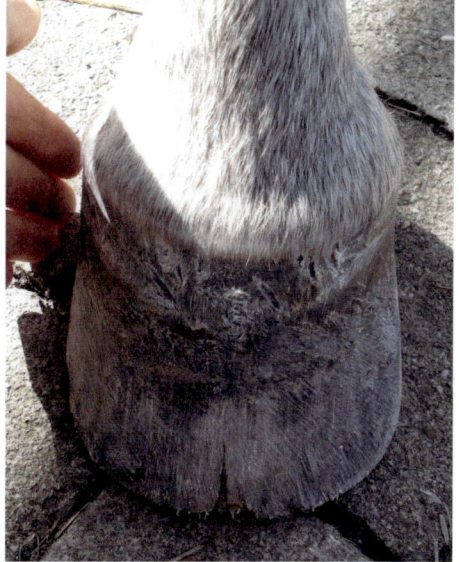

The picture shows the right front hoof (the one with the keratoma) on the 21.7.2009 after a new application with an epoxy resin. Under the translucent resin one can recognize the fiberglass fabric which spans the sandcrack. The fiberglass fabric is double, as also later in the case of acrylic resin.

The hoof on the 14.8.2009, 2 months after the first application, after the previously glued-on fabric had lasted only for 3 ½ weeks (presumably because of unclean working before the gluing) and therefore had to be rasped away. The rasping had led to superficial damages of the horn below the coronet, which could have been avoided!

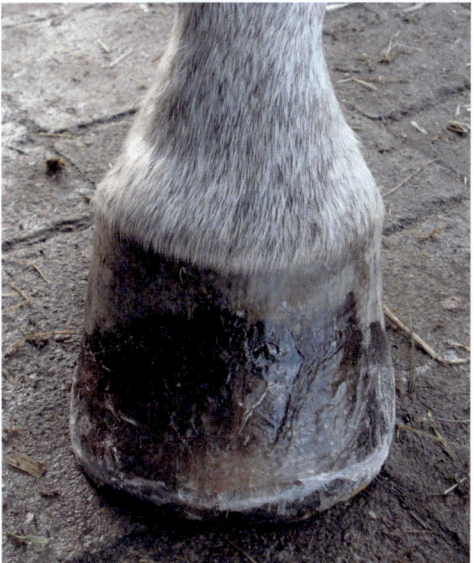

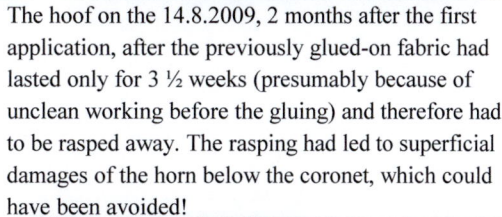

The hoof with an acrylic resin application (16.10.2009). Since this resin is lower-viscous, the layer is thinner.

The hoof on the 22.11.2009. The sandcrack has already almost completely grown-out.

The gluing is done as follows:
- An eventually existing **old layer is rasped off**.
- Afterwards the hoof is **sanded** with an **abrasive paper** at those places, where later is glued-on. (If you only work on the hoof with the rasp, the gluing does not last as long, as when sanding the surface down!)
- **Abrasive dust is wiped off** with a grease-free cloth or paper. (Generally the **hoof** must be **grease-free!)**
- The **fiberglass fabric** is **cut out in the required size**. (Attention, it frays very easily!) For **small horses** use a **double layer**, for **big horses a triple layer is preferable**. If you want to strengthen the hoof wall even more, more layers can be used. For applying a **double layer**, the fiberglass fabric is simply **folded**.
- The **coronet** is protected temporarily from the glue with a **masking tape**, as painters use it for example at windows. (This can already happen before the rasping and protects the coronet!)
- The **acrylic resin** (or another suitable resin with a processing time of about 5 minutes) is prepared **according to the instructions for use**. (The components are mixed in a plastic cup thoroughly.) For mixing and applying the resin you should best wear **disposable gloves**, with which you can touch the liquid resin!
- The mixed, still relatively **low-viscous resin** is **applied** with a flat (e.g. wooden) spatula (or something else lint-free) **onto the sanded hoof wall**, until the whole surface, on which later is glued-on, is impregnated with it.
- The **fiberglass fabric** is **soaked** (in the folded state) with the rest of the still relatively **low-viscous resin** and **placed onto the pre-impregnated hoof**, adjusted and pressed on. Attention, the soaked fiberglass fabric is quite slippery!
- Subsequently, the resin is allowed to **harden**. In summer it is enough to leave the horse tethered for a quarter of an hour, then the gluing is dry to the touch. In **colder weather** (less than 20°C) you can warm the glue with a **hair dryer** for some time, until the glue is hard enough. However, some horses do not like this. It is easier, in my opinion, to cover the not yet hardened resin as a precaution with a thin foil and then to press the **disposable gloves, filled with hot water**, onto the applied layer and leave it there for some time. By this measure the curing is started and within some minutes leads to a sufficient hardening, which allows to roughly rasp the applied layers for a first time to remove protruding parts. The **final rasping** takes place only **the next day after complete hardening**.

As already reported in the preceding chapter, I have continued with the gluing onto the hoof wall on the right keratoma front hoof of my thoroughbred, although the sandcrack has grown out long ago. I would like to recommend this procedure also to others, whose horses have keratomas.

Before trying to eliminate sandcracks by gluing, however, **the utmost must be done to eliminate their causes**! This includes improperly prepared hooves! You should consult a specialist.

But even the specialists do not all work the same way and not all equally well. It is actually surprising that there are so many different methods for preparing hooves, where theoretically there should only be one. And there are always new ones added, e.g. by the Argentinean (of German descent) Daniel Anz, whose method was thoroughly investigated and found to be good by the University of Leipzig.
As remarked in the foreword to the English edition, I now very much prefer this kind of preparing the hooves and advise to use it! (www.f-balance.com)

G. Glued-on dressings above wounds

Wounds on horses are often difficult to dress, especially those on moving parts (joints). The frequently used high bandages from the hoof upwards also hinder the movement of the horse and are therefore sometimes even disadvantageous to healing.
However, in my opinion you should not simply leave wounds, even smaller ones, open. (But you should not worry about the very small ones: the horse's body has to learn how to cope with these injuries itself!)
Especially in summer, flies and dirt that gets into the wound can delay the healing very much and also lead to dangerous infections (phlegmons).
Spray-on dressings or ointments that cover the wound, do not prove successful for every horse.
Already many years ago I have learned from my veterinarian the simple procedure described below, which has since proven very successful! For some time now I have not seen the procedure in use from veterinary side any more! (Probably because it is too easy and too cheap......!)

1.) At first the **wound** is **cleaned**, as usual, and is then treated with an **antiseptic ointment**. (Personally I prefer Furacin® or Tyrosur® gel, but there are certainly also other good ointments. A Microdacyn®-soaked piece of absorbent dressing is also very suitable.)

2.) **At the edges** of a sufficiently sized piece of air-permeable **absorbent gauze** an **all-purpose adhesive** (in Germany I use UHU® Alleskleber) is applied and the **gauze** then **glued directly onto the fur** in safe distance to the wound and the edges are pressed on gently. For this, the gauze should be slightly **gathered**, so that it does not lie directly on the wound and and does not stretch on it when the horse is moving! At moving parts, such as joints, this applies even more, to prevent that tractive forces are exerted on the gluing!

You should not press the glue so firmly onto the fur that it penetrates the fur down to the skin, because otherwise the gauze is loosened only with difficulty later on.

You do not need not remove the dressing every day (of course this depends also on the wound), it is often enough to change the dressing every two to three days. Moreover, it is **often sufficient to loosen only one corner of the glue-on dressing and then to put new ointment onto the wound under it (if necessary).**
Stains of glue on the fur will go away after a while. One should not try to remove them by force!

H. Gentle method of growth inhibition of equine sarcoids

Equine sarcoids are viral skin tumors that occur in different forms. Cause of the tumors are probably mostly bovine papillomaviruses, so actually viruses that come from cattle. For genital sarcoids, a virus specific to horses has also been detected (Equus caballus papillomavirus-2, S. Brandt et al., Equine Veterinary Journal (2010), 42 (8)).
After a treatment / removal, the sarcoid often grows anew. The treatments are sometimes very aggressive and lead to deep wounds.
In contrast to treatment of melanoma, ginger in lower and middle dosages (in any case up to about 12 grams per 100 kilograms of body weight) is is not sufficient for the treatment of this fast-growing and virus-induced tumor. High dosages (more than 25 grams per 100 kilos of body weight) were not tested!
A partial success resulted from the alternating application of cod liver oil and liverwort extract! An enlargement of the sarcoids could thereby be prevented, a very small decrease in size may even have occurred. Skin areas that were already altered, but had not formed a "knob", at least changed their appearance again and became more like normal skin.
The experiment was first carried out over several months only with liverwort extract, which was applied concentrated on the affected skin. Liver moss extract has the effect of reducing the increased growth rate of tumor cells to the normal rate of cell division. This effect was determined in vitro by the son of Prof. Frahm on mouse cancer cells.
Liverwort extract alone, however, showed no observable effect here and the sarcoids continued to grow.
Subsequently, cod liver oil was applied to the affected areas for several weeks. The idea behind it was that cod liver oil has a very high content of vitamin D and vitamin D is known to also slow down tumor growth. However, cod liver oil alone did not show any observable effect.
Thereafter, the treatment was carried out alternately and liverwort extract and cod liver oil were applied alternately. This actually led to a significant effect, in which no growth took place! Unfortunately, though, no healing took place!
However, on sensitive parts of the body or if smaller sarcoids do not disturb and if the horse owner does not mind to have to treat almost every day, this gentle treatment is in my opinion useful in many cases. It has been shown that it is already sufficient to apply liverwort extract on the first day and on the second day cod liver oil and then leave the skin untreated on the third day and only then start again from the beginning.

Appendix exceeding the fourth German edition: At the end I got rid of the sarcoids in a peculiar way: In a winter my thoroughbred got a viral infection from a new horse in the stable and got fever of 39.5 degrees Celsius (103 degrees Fahrenheit). The vet wanted to give something to press the fever down but I refused, because fever has a function in the body and as long as it is not life-threatening and you are careful and cautious, you should not try to decrease it! Though giving no antipyretic drug, the fever was below 39 degrees Celsius (102 degrees Fahrenheit) on the next day and returned to normal 37,5 degrees Celsius (99.5 degrees Fahrenheit) within a week. And with the end of the fever, the sarcoids began to shrink. After several months the knobs were virtually gone and the skin around them started to grow hair again! I stopped the treatment with liverwort extract and cod liver oil and the sarcoids stayed away permanently! In my opinion, the infection and fever killed the bovine papillomavirus and thus the cause for the equine sarcoids!

Hence, if your horse has a strong fever, it can also have an advantage from this!

Healings of this kind are known since a long time, thousands of years! You can read more about about them in Wikipedia under "Coley's toxins", or more informative here:

"Dr William Coley and tumour regression: a place in history or in the future" by S. A. Hoption Cann, J. P. van Netten, C. van Netten

https://www.ncbi.nlm.nih.gov/pubmed/14707241

https://www.ncbi.nlm.nih.gov/pmc/articles/PMC1742910/pdf/v079p00672.pdf

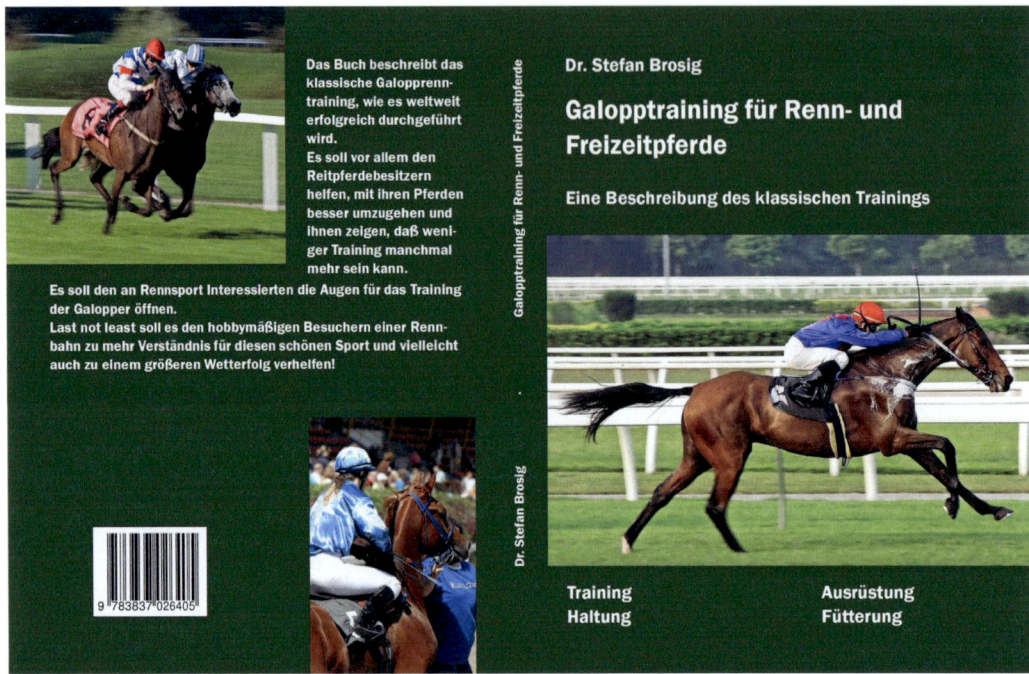

Das Buch beschreibt das klassische Galopprenntraining, wie es weltweit erfolgreich durchgeführt wird.
Es soll vor allem den Reitpferdebesitzern helfen, mit ihren Pferden besser umzugehen und ihnen zeigen, daß weniger Training manchmal mehr sein kann.
Es soll den an Rennsport Interessierten die Augen für das Training der Galopper öffnen.
Last not least soll es den hobbymäßigen Besuchern einer Rennbahn zu mehr Verständnis für diesen schönen Sport und vielleicht auch zu einem größeren Wetterfolg verhelfen!

Galopptraining für Renn- und Freizeitpferde

Dr. Stefan Brosig

Dr. Stefan Brosig

Galopptraining für Renn- und Freizeitpferde

Eine Beschreibung des klassischen Trainings

Training   **Ausrüstung**
Haltung   **Fütterung**

9 783837 026405

Only in German language!

For centuries, the knowledge of the classic training of the racehorse has only been passed on by word of mouth, from the coach to his jockeys and apprentices, who in turn passed them on to their own jockeys and trainees during their own trainer's life.

More literature can be found about interval training methods, which were modern in the US for some time. The classical training, as it developed empirically over the centuries and which, with slight deviations, is performed worldwide, however, is exhaustively written down nowhere. This book wants to help close this gap. It is based on a training course at the German Directorate for Thoroughbred Breeding and Racing, but often refers to the experiences of Germany's most successful gallop race trainer, Heinz Jentzsch.

The book also helps owners of riding horses to train their horses better.

Contents: Thoroughbred breeding / The races / Keeping / Feed / Shoeing of the racehorse / Exterior / Coat color and performance / The equipment of horse and rider in the race / Stable routines: One working day in the stable / Training: / A. Flat racing / Training basics / Comparison of training with humans and horses / Overview of the general training procedure / Training of three-year-old and older horses / Preparation of the yearling / Training of the two-year-old / B. Hurdle Racing / General / Training / Doping / Genetics / Explanation of racing terms / A racehorse as a riding horse? Tips for buying / Attachments: / Quick guide for feeding of ginger to horses / Quick guide for feeding of horseradish to horses / Analysis of energy consumption in the movement of the racehorse

Available through the book trade ISBN: 978-3-8370-2640-5
(Price in Germany 18.90 Euro, BoD-Verlag, 164 pages, format 17 x 22 cm)